Soyfoods Cooking
for a
Positive
Menopause

Bryanna Clark Grogan

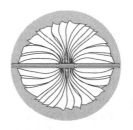

Book Publishing Company
Summertown, Tennessee

© 1999 Bryanna Clark Grogan
Cover design: Studio Haus
Cover photos: © 1999 PhotoDisk, Inc.
Interior design: Warren Jefferson
Editor: Karen Sullivan

Published in the United States of America by:

Book Publishing Co.
P.O. Box 99
Summertown, TN 38483
888-260-8458

04 03 02 01 00 99   6 5 4 3 2 1

ISBN 1-57067-067-5

Grogan, Bryanna Clark
    Soyfoods cooking for a positive menopause / Bryanna Clark Grogan.
            p.   cm.
    Includes bibliographical references and index.
    ISBN 1-57067-076-5 (alk. paper)
    1. Menopause--Complications--Diet therapy. 2. Soyfoods-
    -Therapeutic use. 3. Cookery (Soybeans)   I. Title.
RG186.G76 1999
618.1'750654--dc21   99-39151
                                                CIP

Calculations for the nutritional analyses in this book are based on the average number of servings listed with the recipes and the average amount of an ingredient, if a range is called for. Calculations are rounded up to the nearest gram. If two options for an ingredient are listed, the first one is used. Not included are optional ingredients, serving suggestions, or fat used for frying, unless the amount of fat is specified in the recipe.

This book is for my mother, Eve Tonge Urbina.

Thanks to the soy pioneers: William Shurtleff,
Akiko Aoyagi, Virginia Messina, Mark
Messina, and Kenneth Setchell, who gave the
North American public a new awareness of
the goodness of soy.

Table of Contents

Introduction

The good news about menopause

"Good news?" you ask. "Is there any *good* news about menopause?" We are constantly bombarded by negative images of female aging. Menopausal women are the butt of jokes, and "the change" is blamed for everything from being out of sorts or in a crazy mood to severe depression.

It may surprise you to learn that in other cultures women look forward to the change of life. Postmenopausal women in many other cultures enjoy the status of elders in their communities, respected for their wisdom and experience. They look forward to a sex life unencumbered by the possibility of pregnancy. Mayan women in Mexico interviewed about their attitudes toward menopause consistently referred to feeling like young girls again because of their newfound freedom. They don't understand the Western concept of menopause as an "endocrine deficiency disease," and they're not familiar with hot flashes and other common Western menopausal discomforts.

Japanese women have no word for hot flash, and only a small percentage of them describe having any discomforts even vaguely like night sweats, major sleep disturbances, or hot flashes. Filipino women look forward to the joys of old age, to being loved and respected by not only their family, but by society in general. In many Asian and aboriginal cultures, postmenopausal woman are held in high esteem and expected to be vital and productive into old age, with many native herbal remedies available to them if they should experience unpleasant discomforts.

Unfortunately, in most Western cultures the prevailing attitude seems to be that we will "dry up" (I can't tell you how many times I've heard this particular phrase in relation to older women!), lose our sexuality, become depressed or hysterical, and rapidly lose bone mass until we have to retire to an old-age home and spend our days in front of a TV—unless we take estrogen-replacement therapy for the rest of our lives to remedy the "deficiency disease" of aging!

As I enter my 50s, a proud grandmother of granddaughters Savannah, Kate, Hannah, and Mariah, and grandson, Levon, I'm happy to report that I'm slimmer and more physically fit than I have been for years. I continue to work and to learn; this is my fifth book in six years, and I began

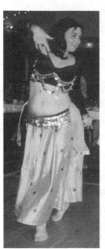

to study belly dancing two years ago. I am in excellent health, with strong muscles and bones. I have no hot flashes, night sweats, sleep disturbances, depression, mental lapses, or other common Western menopausal discomforts. And my libido is just fine, thank you very much!

I believe that I am experiencing what Margaret Mead called "postmenopausal zest," a time when many women experience vastly increased stores of energy. And it is an exciting time to experience this, along with so many sister baby boomers: vital, outspoken, active, innovative women who reject the negative images of aging and celebrate their "cronehood": maturity and age of wisdom. No sweeping "the change" under the carpet for this generation! We are taking control of our bodies in a new way—no longer concerned with reproductive freedom, but with living happy, healthy, and creative lives into old age. We no longer accept whatever the doctor, however well intentioned, tells us. We demand accurate information so that we can make our own decisions about our futures, and we seek out the experiences and expertise of the grandmothers and sisters in older—and, in some ways, wiser—cultures.

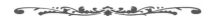

Due to endometriosis, I had a complete hysterectomy at age 37, when the youngest of my four children was about 9 years old. I did not take estrogen-replacement therapy (ERT) for a few years, because my doctor advised me to wait until I experienced any discomforts and then decide. Eventually, hot flashes, night sweats, and concern about osteoporosis and heart disease convinced me to take a very low dose of synthetic estrogen for approximately eight years.

I decided to discontinue estrogen-replacement therapy cold turkey in late 1997, when my chiropractor suggested that it might be exacerbating the migraine headaches I'd had since I was a teenager. The difference was so dramatic that I have been headache-free for the first time since I was about 16. I do not intend ever to resume taking ERT.

I expected some hot flashes and other problems after so abruptly discontinuing ERT; in fact, many health practitioners recommend a more gradual cessation. But I had only mild and infrequent hot flashes for a few months. When I thought about why I had such an easy transition, I realized that I had drastically changed my diet in the previous ten years. I went from a health food-style omnivorous diet to semivegetarianism, then full-fledged vegetarianism, and finally to low-fat veganism with a lot of soy products.

Soy just happens to be one of the best natural sources of phytochemicals, natural compounds in plants that include antioxidants and plant-based estrogens, which appear to protect not only against common menopausal discomforts but also the number one killer of North American women: heart disease. Phytochemicals also may ward off osteoporosis, stroke, breast cancer, and other diseases that plague postmenopausal women in the Western world.

I believe that my soy-rich diet, along with exercise, eased my body's reaction to the abrupt cessation of ERT and let me sail through what Gail Sheehy, author of *The Silent Passage: Menopause*, calls the "menopause gateway" into the postmenopausal period that she terms "coalescence: a time when all the wisdom a woman has gathered from fifty years of experience in living comes together."

In this book, I'd like to share, in layperson's terms, what I have learned about soy products—how they may ease you through your "menopause gateway" and help you retain your health and zest for living in the postmenopausal years.

And, by the way, this is not an anti-estrogen book. I know that it can be very helpful for some women who have tried every possible natural therapy without relief for very severe discomforts. But I have strong concerns about the advisability of taking estrogen past the usual time of menopause, around age 50, and I believe that women need as much information as possible to make an intelligent choice. While it is beyond the scope of this book to recommend specific therapies, the bibliography on page 178 lists resources where you can get more information.

Soyfoods eaten daily as part of a low-fat, plant-based diet, along with regular vigorous exercise, can bring us closest to the traditional lifestyle of Asian women, who are physically active and eat a diet rich in antioxidants and plant estrogens. If discomforts persist, intelligent use of certain vitamins and herbal preparations can be combined with diet and exercise. Given the very real concerns about breast, uterine, and endometrial cancer that accompany every decision to take hormone or estrogen replacement therapy, and the many other ways that a low-fat, plant-based diet has been medically proven to enhance our health, this type of approach should certainly be made known to and considered by every woman.

Even without soy, a plant-based diet can still be protective. The Mayan women I spoke of earlier don't eat soy, but their traditional diet is low in meat and dairy, as are most Oriental diets, and high in plant foods, including the wild yam from which many natural hormone products are derived. These yams also contain plant estrogens and antioxidants. They ingest large quantities of calcium not in milk products or tofu, but in corn tortillas, which are made from corn processed with calcium in the form of lime. However, for our Western diet, it is easier to incorporate soy into our favorite foods every day than to depend on plants for phytoestrogens, since we have very little data on how much each plant contains. Soyfoods have been intensely studied, so we know the quantity of phytoestrogens contained in various common soy products, and most are versatile enough to be used in familiar North American dishes instead of dairy products or meat.

Because I'm a cookbook writer, I'd like to share my favorite soy recipes and some ideas for painlessly incorporating soy into your daily diet. You may find that you enjoy some of the traditional Asian ways of eating soyfoods, or you may prefer a more Westernized approach. You may decide to use one or two soyfoods in the same way every day, for instance, switching from milk to soymilk on your cereal and a having a tofu-fruit shake after your walk or run. Or you might instead eat a variety of soyfoods in new and exciting ways every day. Whichever way you prefer, I feel sure that within these covers you will find some helpful ideas and delicious recipes that suit you.

Bryanna Clark Grogan

Glossary

Here are some terms you will need to know. Please read through this list of definitions before reading the following chapters, and refer back to it as you read. Let's start with some basic terms you'll see over and over:

Estrogen: a class of hormones important in promoting female characteristics. Men also produce them, but in smaller amounts.

Free radicals: Unstable oxygen molecules produced by normal metabolism that can damage normal cells. They are regulated by enzymes called antioxidants (or free-radical scavengers) and other substances such as phytochemicals found in the body. Free radicals are also produced in response to radiation and industrial pollution. Free radical damage is thought to be responsible, at least in part, for a wide range of diseases, including heart disease and cancer, as well as normal symptoms of aging.

Hormone: produced by living cells, it is a chemical substance circulating in the body fluids that produces a specific effect on the activity of cells. Hormones control blood sugar levels, insulin levels, menstrual cycles, and growth.

Isoflavones: compounds found in plant foods, such as soy, that resemble and act like natural estrogens produced in the body. Many of these compounds are believed to protect against cancer. Also called plant estrogens or phytoestrogens.

Menopause: cessation of menstrual cycles.

Phytochemicals: Compounds found in plant foods that may protect against disease (often referred to as nutriceuticals). Some phytochemicals are called antioxidants and protect cells from free radicals; others deactivate carcinogens or boost the immune system.

Phytoestrogen: A compound structurally similar to human estrogen that binds with estrogen receptors in the human body. Phytoestrogens are believed to protect against breast and prostate cancers, two hormone-dependent cancers. *See isoflavones.*

Here are some other terms you'll want to be familiar with:

Antioxidant: a chemical compound, or type of phytochemical, that neutralizes cell-damaging free radicals created when oxygen is used inside the body's cells. Antioxidants appear to have a protective effect against cancer, heart disease, other degenerative diseases, and symptoms of aging. The main antioxidants are beta-carotene, vitamins C and E, and the trace mineral selenium. However, scientists have not yet isolated or discovered all of the antioxidants, so it is best to depend on foods, not supplements, as sources. Plant foods, particularly brightly colored fruits and vegetables, all contain antioxidants. Legumes, including soybeans, are good sources too.

Daidzein: a powerful isoflavone in soybeans. Shown to have anticarcinogenic properties, and may also have bone-building properties.

Equol: an estrogenic-like compound that intestinal bacteria produce from isoflavones. Found in the urine of people who eat soy.

ERT (estrogen replacement therapy): the most common type of prescription estrogen therapy. Uses only estrogen, and no progesterone or progestin. Most often prescribed for women who have had hysterectomies, because progesterone or progestin are thought to be protective against uterine cancer and are not necessary for a woman who has had her uterus removed.

Estradiol (E2): the most common estrogen found circulating in the blood stream in premenopausal women.

Estriol (E3): produced in largest amounts during pregnancy, it is the weakest of the primary human estrogens.

Estrone (E1): the most common estrogen found circulating in the blood stream in postmenopausal women. May be linked to increased risk of endometrial cancer (in the mucous-membrane lining of the uterus) and breast cancer.

FSH (follicle stimulating hormone): At the beginning of a woman's monthly cycle, the pituitary gland releases FSH. This stimulates the ovaries to develop and enlarge several follicles, which contain egg cells.

Genistein: an isoflavone found exclusively in soyfoods that has been shown in laboratory studies to inhibit the growth of both breast cancer and prostate cancer cells. It has also been shown to convert cancer cells into normal cells, thus preventing the spread of the cancer.

HDL (high-density lipoprotein): sometimes called "good" cholesterol because it is the body's major carrier of cholesterol to the liver for excretion in the bile. The ratio between total cholesterol and HDL should not exceed 6:1.

HRT (hormone replacement therapy): the administration of hormones when there is no longer enough being produced by the body in sufficient quantities to maintain regular periods. The most common form, prescribed for women who have not had a hysterectomy, is generally a combination of estrogen and progesterone or progestin. The latter two are thought to be protective against uterine cancer.

LDL (low-density lipoprotein): sometimes referred to as "bad" cholesterol, these proteins carry cholesterol through the bloodstream. Studies show that high levels of LDL increase the risk of heart disease.

Legumes: a plant food group containing protein-rich green peas and beans, and dried beans such as soybeans, lentils, kidney beans, and split peas.

LH (luteinizing hormone): produced by the pituitary gland. When combined with FSH, the two stimulate the ovary to secrete estrogen and begin ovulation. It is also responsible for the development of the corpus luteum, the progesterone-producing sac that is formed within the ovary from the remains of the follicle after the release of the egg. LH levels rise dramatically during menopause and stay elevated throughout postmenopause. This is thought to have something to do with the occurrence of hot flashes.

mg/dl: milligrams per deciliter.

Nutriceutical: nutritional substance produced from foods that is deemed to have benefits to health but is not considered a drug or nutrient, such as soy protein. See phytochemicals.

Omega-3 and omega-6 fatty acids: natural substances found in various oils that may lower the risk of heart disease and may help prevent cancer. They are called "essential fatty acids," because the body cannot produce them; they must be obtained from the foods we eat. Although fish oil has been promoted as the best source of omega-3s, full-fat soy products are one of the few plant sources that are rich in them.

Perimenopause or premenopause: the time before menopause when hormonal changes begin to occur and periods may become irregular. Bone loss may increase, and menopausal discomforts such as sleep disturbance and hot flashes may occur. Perimenopause can occur at different ages for different women.

Phenolic acids: a class of antioxidant that may prevent DNA from being attacked by harmful carcinogens.

Phytic acid, phytate: an antioxidant compound found in soy and other plant foods that has been shown to inhibit tumor growth in animals, especially colon and breast cancers.

Phyto-: denotes a relationship to plants.

Phytohormone: a hormone found in plants. These may help prevent heart disease by moving cholesterol out of the body quickly, and may help prevent colon and skin cancers. Phytohormone intake is highest in populations with low rates of colon cancer—the Japanese, vegetarians, and Seventh Day Adventists.

Phytosterol: used interchangeably with phytohormone.

Postmenopause: the years after cessation of menstruation.

Progesterone: a natural ovarian hormone made by the corpus luteum (see LH) to sustain the endometrium (mucous membrane lining of the uterus) and support the fertilized egg.

Progestin: a synthetic form of progesterone (medroxy-progesterone acetate or megestrol acetate); also known as progestogen in England, and gestogen in Europe.

Prostaglandins: chemicals composed of fatty acids that have a hormone-like effect. They influence muscular contractions, circulation, and inflammation. They can regulate cell behavior and inhibit hormones.

Protease inhibitors: plant compounds that inhibit the action of certain enzymes that promote the growth of tumors; known as the universal anticarcinogen.

Saponins: a type of antioxidant; compounds derived from sugars that occur in many plant, but not animal, proteins. Characterized by their ability to foam in water (hence the appropriately named soapberry, which Native Americans beat into frothy desserts), they also have been found to possess an anti-inflammatory action similar to that of cortisone. Once thought to be harmful, they are now thought to lower cholesterol and may also be anticarcinogenic. Soyfoods are rich in saponins, which are also found in herbs long used in folk medicines, such as goldenrod, ginseng, chickweed, and wild yam, and in other legumes and seeds.

Soy protein isolate: a concentrated soy product that contains no less than 90 percent protein. Also contains isoflavones and phytates.

Testosterone: the major male sex hormone produced in the testes; also produced in smaller amounts by the ovaries of women.

Chapter 1

The soy prescription for menopause

It's hard to make the humble soybean sexy, in the advertising copywriter's parlance. It's pretty unprepossessing—small, hard, and beige, with a flavor that doesn't exactly say "wow!" Oh, sure, mainstream magazines have caught on to the fact that soy is a nutritional powerhouse with all kinds of health benefits, and they'll offer a few low-key soy recipes. Even gourmet magazines run the occasional tofu article these days. But I get the feeling that they aren't taking soy really *seriously*—it just doesn't have the pizzazz of gourmet superstars like sun-dried tomatoes, chili peppers, and balsamic vinegar, or the Mediterranean health trio of garlic, wine, and olive oil.

But under that unassuming Clark Kent exterior, the soybean is a sexy superbean! After all, it's chock-full of plant hormones—phytoestrogens called isoflavones—that are constructed very much like the female sex hormone estrogen. These phytoestrogens have all sorts of potential health benefits—from decreasing cholesterol to preventing hot flashes—and none of the potentially harmful side effects of wine and olive oil, such as addiction problems, cancer risk, and weight gain.

Furthermore, the soybean can be made into a number of delicious and versatile foods that can fit into any healthful cuisine or dietary plan. It's inexpensive and highly nutritious. It contains virtually no saturated fat, but does have essential fatty acids. It's been proven to lower cholesterol levels and decrease risk of heart attack and stroke. It has anticarcinogenic properties and the potential to protect against diabetes, osteoporosis, digestive tract problems, gallstones, kidney disorders, and high blood pressure. It's easy and cheap to grow in a number of climates and soils, and its cultivation adds nutrients to the soil instead of depleting it. Being a high-protein food that's low on the food chain, the soybean has the potential to solve world food shortages. *And* it has potential benefits for menopausal women! Move over, Superman!

This has got to be a miracle food, right? Wrong. There are no miracle foods. Oat bran (remember oat bran?) is a good food, but it wasn't the "roto-rooter" for arteries that it was claimed to be. It couldn't overcome a daily barrage of saturated fats. Neither can olive oil, garlic, wine, or soy products. But given the profile of the soybean, it's easy to see why some health reporters get a little carried away.

Just remember that soyfoods can be a component of what nutritionists, even the nonvegetarians, have to concede is the most healthful style of eating: a plant-based diet containing large amounts of vegetables, grains (including breads and pasta), fruits, beans and other dried legumes, and a few nuts and seeds, with animal foods kept to a minimum or not used at all. This plant-based diet can be adapted to any culinary tradition, whether Mediterranean, Asian, or good old North American. The world of plant foods is so varied that the possibilities for good eating are endless. The soybean's versatility can only add to these possibilities.

That said, what exactly can this sexy little bean do for "women of a certain age"?

Until recently it was the common wisdom that up to 80 percent of menopausal women would experience hot flashes, which menopause expert Fredi Kronenberg defines as recurrent, transient periods of flushing, sweating, and a sensation of heat, often accompanied by palpitations and a feeling of anxiety, and sometimes followed by chills. It turns out that this figure may be highly exaggerated, however. Anthropologist Patricia Kaufert has concluded that much of our information is based on women who have had hysterectomies, which produces an artificially induced, and often instant, menopause and women at special clinics for patients with severe menopause problems. Her own research of midlife women in Manitoba and Massachusetts, conducted with fellow anthropologist Sonja McKinlay, found that only 31 percent and 35 percent of the respondents, respectively, reported hot flashes.

Every woman should be thoroughly informed about the process of menopause and all of the ways that we can help ourselves remain healthy and vital. We need to question our doctors' recommendations for HRT and ERT, because there may be less risky, more natural therapies for women with severe discomforts that are just as effective. (See the bibliography, page 178.)

Some cultures don't even have a word for hot flash. In Japan, McGill University researcher Margaret Locke studied middle-aged women for her book *Encounters with Aging: Mythologies of Menopause in Japan and North America* (University of California Press, 1993). She found that only 10 percent of the women in her study reported anything resembling hot flashes.

Marcha Flint and Ratna Suprapti Samil studied women in India and Indonesia, Y. Beyene studied Mayan women, and Pranee L. Rice studied Hmong women in Southeast Asia. The experience of menopause in all of these cultures was very different from the one that Western women expect. Although cultural expectations and genetic factors may have something to do with this, it does not explain the vast difference in the incidence of physical discomforts in menopausal Asian and North American women. California breast surgeon Robert Kradjian, author of *Save Yourself from Breast Cancer* (Berkeley Books, 1994), says bluntly that "women are biologically the same no matter where in the world they live."

My friend Susan-Marie Yoshihara, in a research paper for the University of Victoria, B. C., Canada, entitled "Hot Flashes, Tofu, and Meno-pause in Japan," effectively demolishes the idea that a relaxed lifestyle might be the explanation for lack of menopausal discomforts by painting a realistic picture of the average middle-aged Japanese woman. Her life is every bit, if not much more, stressful than a North American woman's. She is "absolutely accountable for all domestic, financial, and child raising responsibilities," Yoshihara writes. She usually lives in a tiny house or apartment, which is hot in the summer and cold in the winter, with a minute refrigerator, necessitating daily or twice-daily grocery shopping by foot or bicycle. Child care is virtually nonexistent, and Japanese sarari-man (salaried men) spend little time with their families because of the cultural expectation that they will put their companies before everything. Many midlife women, particularly the wife of the oldest son in a family, have the further responsibility of caring for their aging in-laws; it is so shameful to put them in a nursing home that the family would have to be at the breaking point before this would happen. *Relaxed* would hardly be the word to describe the life of most menopausal Japanese women!

> ### What's a serving of soy?
>
> *One serving of soy contains about 40 milligrams (mg) of isoflavones. Many experts believe that it is better to obtain isoflavones from foods, instead of isolated in pills or supplemental foods, because it isn't known yet whether other components of foods have an effect on the way isoflavones work in the body. Here's what counts as a serving of soy:*
>
> *1 cup regular or low-fat soymilk*
> *¼ cup unreconstituted textured soy protein*
> *4 ounces firm tofu (about ½ cup)*
> *3 ounces extra-firm or pressed tofu*
> *½ cup cooked or raw soybeans*
> *4 ounces tempeh*
> *¾ cup soy yogurt*
> *⅓ cup roasted soybeans (soynuts)*
> *¼ cup soy flour*

Migration studies of other women's health issues, such as breast cancer and osteoporosis, show that place of residence is a stronger predictor of disease than place of birth or racial origin. For instance, Japanese people who live outside Japan and have adopted Western-style eating habits develop these conditions at a much higher rate than those who keep a traditional table regardless of where they are.

A traditional Japanese diet is high in carbohydrates such as rice and noodles, vegetables, and sea vegetables, and very low in fats; fewer than 15 percent of calories come from fat. The traditional diet contains only minute quantities of animal foods, and no dairy products. Soyfoods are featured heavily in the Japanese diet. Hot fresh soymilk might be purchased at a local shop for breakfast. Soup with tofu and miso (fermented soybean paste) is another common breakfast item. Natto, a sticky fermented soybean product, often accompanies the breakfast rice. Other meals of the day contain tofu and miso as well, and boiled, salted fresh green soybeans are a popular snack.

Other cultures in Asia, such as Indonesia, also eat soy products. But the common factor in the diets of these women is a heavy dependence on a large variety of plant foods. We may think of our diet as diverse, but these traditional diets use a vast number of plant foods that we have never even heard of. Many of these plant foods, including the soybean, contain substances called isoflavones, plant estrogens that have been shown to have a mildly estrogen-like effect.

How many servings do you need?

Most experts agree that two to five servings of soy per day are enough to lower cholesterol levels. (See "What's a Serving of Soy?," on the facing page.) Three to eight portions are recommended for protecting bones and easing menopausal discomforts.

Scientists believe that soy isoflavones, a unique group of phytoestrogens found in soy products, can help reduce hot flashes and night sweats by making the menopausal drop in estrogen production more gradual. As a woman approaches menopause, her FSH (follicle-stimulating hormone) levels will rise as the ovaries become more resistant to stimulation. Another hormone, LH (luteinizing hormone), which works in concert with FSH, also rises at the same time. Sudden high levels of LH are known to occur at the beginning of a hot flash. A nine-month study reported in the *British Journal of Nutrition* in 1995 found that levels of the two hormones did not rise as high in premenopausal women who consumed 60 grams of textured soy protein per day. There are now studies underway to test the effects of isoflavones on hot flashes and night sweats.

Isoflavones resemble human estrogens just enough to be accepted by estrogen receptors on cells in the body and bind weakly to the cell surface membrane. The estrogen receptors have been compared to tiny switching stations, locks, or docking stations on the cells. Joanna Dwyer and colleagues at the New England Medical Center and Tufts University theorized in an article they wrote for *The Journal of The American Dietetic Association* (July 1994) that in premenopausal women the estrogen receptors are occupied, and the weaker plant estrogens must compete for these sites. However, in postmenopausal women, whose self-produced estrogen declines about 60 percent, there is a far greater chance of the plant estrogens docking, and this can increase the amount of estrogens available to her, thus decreasing the severity of menopausal discomforts as her body produces less and less estogen.

Perhaps the most important soybean estrogen is an isoflavone called *genistein*. It is considered a powerful anticarcinogen (see page 9) and is found in good supply in whole soybeans, including roasted soybeans or soynuts, textured soy protein, soy flour, soymilk, tofu and tofu products, and tempeh. *Daidzein*, another isoflavone generously supplied by these soy foods, is now under intense study for its potential cancer-fighting and bone-building qualities. Intestinal bacteria turn it, as well as genistein, into a substance that can act as a weak form of human estrogen. Although other foods contain plant hormones, *no other commonly consumed foods contain these two powerful phytoestrogens*. And it has been proven in human studies that isoflavones in the diet are absorbed into the bloodstream, thus making them available for assimilation by the body. In one study where volunteers ate 40 grams of textured soy protein daily for just five days, the isoflavone levels in their urine (which indicates their presence in the bloodstream) increased as much as one thousand times compared to levels taken before the study.

In fact, in a 1993 study, women who ate soy for two months had an average increase of two and a half days in the length of their menstrual cycles, which attests to the powerful effect phytoestrogens can have on a woman's body.

Soy may also prove to be "sexy" in another way, by preventing the thinning of the vaginal walls, a common condition in menopause that can cause painful intercourse and may contribute to infections. A study reported in the *British Medical Journal* in 1990 found that when post-menopausal women were given soy flour every day for two weeks, the number of cells in the vaginal lining increased compared to two week periods during which they were given flaxseed oil or red clover sprouts instead of the soy flour (as these foods also contain phytoestrogens).

Of course, eating soyfoods is not the only thing you can do for common menopausal discomforts. There are other natural remedies that work well for many women, such as taking herbs like black cohosh (a common brand is Remifemin); taking nutritional supplements, such as the antioxidant vitamins C (very helpful for hot flashes!), E, and beta-carotene; eating a low-fat, high-fiber plant-based diet; exercising often; and doing strength training. *But adding soy to your diet may be the only thing that you need to do, so why not try it first?* It can certainly be, at the very least, a component of your own personal menopause program, and it promises many other benefits for women's health, as well as for the men in their lives, as you will learn in the following chapters.

What About Soy Isolates?

Soy protein isolate can contain 15 to 103 mg of isoflavones per ounce. The wide variation is due to a number of factors, including the type of soybeans used, the climate they were grown in, etc., and standards and procedures for measuring the isoflavone content of foods are still being determined. Some manufacturers will list the average isoflavone content of their product on the label. Solgar Iso-Soy Powder, GeniSoy UltraSoy Protein Powder, and Take Care Soy Protein Powder all list high levels of isoflavones. Tests are being done now on the isoflavone content of meat analogs. Some experts say that you can count one soyburger or two soy hot dogs as a soy serving, but the isoflavone content isn't certain yet. Don't depend on soy oil, soy cheese, soy sauce, soy bacon bits, tofu yogurt powders, or miso for isoflavones. Miso, for instance, contains about 40 mg per ½ cup, but that is a lot of miso for one person to eat!

Chapter 2

Soy for strong bones and weight loss

I don't know many women who *aren't* worried about osteoporosis, which is Latin for porous or spongy bones and is also known as brittle-bone disease. Some women are following doctor's orders and guzzling glasses of skim milk daily or popping calcium pills morning, noon, and night. Some are taking up walking, running, and weight lifting. Some are considering estrogen or hormone replacement therapy. A surprising number are doing little more than worry, confused by all the conflicting information.

Scientists can't agree on whether this degenerative condition is a disease of deficiency or a disease of excess. They can't agree on how much calcium we need or where we should be getting it. The only thing they do agree on is that this disease is of epidemic proportions, with experts estimating that one in three North American women will develop it. This disease is more than a cosmetic problem of the unsightly "dowager's hump." Osteoporosis can cause extreme discomfort and even death, and the statistics are frightening. The average North American woman will have lost more than one-third of her skeletal structure by age 65! In severe cases of osteoporosis, bones fracture spontaneously because they can't support the body's weight. The impact of a sneeze can splinter small bones.

While 80 percent of sufferers are women, men are not immune. More men will get osteoporosis than prostate cancer. However, men have a larger bone mass to start with, giving them an advantage, and they do not experience the accelerated bone loss of 3 or more percent each year during the first seven to ten years after menopause that women do. Men have an average yearly bone loss of 1 percent after age 50. Women generally return to this rate after the years of rapid loss.

Rates of hip fracture, a common result of osteoporosis, are used as a measure of the disease. Hip fractures are the number one reason for winding up in a nursing home these days. Half of these hip fracture patients will be temporarily or permanently disabled, and 20 percent will die within one year. And things are getting worse every year.

How can this be in North America, where people drink milk by the gallon, yogurt is a popular snack and breakfast food, and cheese consumption has been increasing? Everybody knows that you can prevent osteoporosis if you get enough calcium, and aren't these dairy products chock-full of calcium?

Well, it's a little more complicated than we've been led to believe. The diet of North Americans tends to be high in animal protein, phosphorous, and sodium. These all cause the body to lose calcium through the urine. Thus, North American women need to consume much more calcium just to maintain their calcium balance and bone health than women in developing nations, who eat far less of these things. The common recommendation by the USDA to eat 1,000 milligrams (mg) of calcium per day presumes that you'll also be eating four ounces of animal protein a day; in addition, for every ounce of animal protein over four ounces, you need an extra 100 mg of calcium.

But unfortunately, ingesting higher levels of calcium does not necessarily compensate for calcium loss. If osteoporosis were merely a deficiency disease, then we should be seeing rates of osteoporosis in North America and other milk-consuming, calcium-supplement-popping areas of the world go down—but they are going up! In fact, the hip-fracture rates go up as consumption of calcium goes up (see chart below). Paradoxically, countries with the lowest rates of calcium intake also have the lowest rates of hip fracture.

In fact, the World Health Organization recommends that adults in developing countries consume between 400 and 500 mg of calcium per day. In Japan, which has less osteoporosis than North America even though Asians' bones are less dense than those of Caucasians, the recommended daily dose of calcium is 600 mg, but the actual intakes are probably half that. In North America, adult women are advised by the WHO to take between 800 and 1,500 mg a day.

ANIMAL PROTEIN AND CALCIUM INTAKE AND HIP-FRACTURE RATES			
Population	Av. Daily Calcium	Av. Daily Animal Protein	Rate of Hip Fracture/ 100,000
S. African Blacks	196 mg	10.4 g	6.8
Singapore	389 mg	24.7 g	21.7
Yugoslavia	588 mg	27.3 g	27.6
U.S.	973 mg	56.6 g	144.9
Norway	1,087 mg	66.6 g	190.4
Source: The Simple Soybean and Your Health, by Messina & Messina			

According to Virginia Messina, a registered dietician with a master's degree in public health, and Mark Messina, Ph.D., formerly with the Diet and Cancer Branch of the National Cancer Institute in the United States, writing in their book *The Vegetarian Way* (Crown Trade Paperbacks, 1996): "Osteoporosis, like heart disease, cancer, diabetes, and obesity, appears to a be a disease of affluence and excess, rather than one of deficiency. The more scientists learn about osteoporosis, the more they realize that it is an extremely complex disease related to overall lifestyle, a big part of which includes diet. The idea that dosing yourself with calcium will automatically keep your bones in good shape is just plain wrong."

They go on to say further "that the belief that milk is essential in the diet is clearly incorrect," given that about two-thirds of the world's population has trouble digesting milk. Anthropologists tell us that apparently northern Europeans developed a genetic mutation that allows them to digest milk sugar into adulthood. Populations throughout the rest of the world, including Asians, Native Americans, Africans, and Mediterraneans, lose this ability as they mature. It is obvious that drinking milk is not taking calcium the way nature intended it.

Now, consider this statement from the most recent position paper of the American Dietetic Association on vegetarian diets: "Calcium absorption appears to be inhibited by such plant constituents as phytic acid, oxalic acid, and fiber, but this effect may not be significant. Calcium deficiency in vegetarians is rare, and there is little evidence to show that low intakes of calcium give rise to major health problems among the vegetarian population. One recent study has shown that vegetarians absorb and retain more calcium from foods than do nonvegetarians. Other studies cite lower rates of osteoporosis in vegetarians than in nonvegetarians."

The operative words here appear to be *absorb* and *retain*. Ingesting huge quantities of calcium seems to be of little use if they are not absorbed and retained by the body. Scientists are discovering that many factors influence the way the body absorbs calcium, and that the calcium in foods is not all equally well absorbed. One of the problems in our North American diet appears to be an excess of animal protein. Consider that at age 65 female vegetarians have an average measurable bone loss of only 7 percent, compared to the 35 percent average.

The protein connection

As far back as the 1930s, researchers noted that a meat-based diet caused large increases in the amount of calcium excreted in the urine. More current studies have found that the more protein consumed, the more calcium is lost from the body. Increasing total protein from 48 grams a day (just a bit below the recommended dietary allowance, or RDA) to 95 grams a day (the amount consumed by the average North American) causes a *50 percent increase* in the amount of calcium excreted. When the amount of protein in the diet is very high at 142 grams a day (common in North America) *it is impossible to maintain calcium balance, even when ingesting 1,400 mg of calcium a day.*

How does this happen? To state it very simply, consuming a lot of protein creates an acidic condition that the body attempts to bring back into balance by leaching calcium, an alkaline mineral, from the bones. One extreme example of this is Inuit people on a traditional meat-and-fish-based diet with few plant foods. They consume some of the highest amounts of calcium in the world—more than 2,000 mg a day—but also eat very high amounts of protein, about 250 to 400 grams a day. They have one of the highest rates of osteoporosis in the world.

By contrast, traditional African Bantu women consume a low-protein, low-calcium (350 mg a day) diet, mostly vegetables and grains. Yet even the oldest women are essentially free of osteoporosis. Genetic relatives of these women who live in the United States and eat the standard North American diet have the same rate of osteoporosis as the average American woman.

John McDougall, M.D., an authority on diet and disease, writes: " I would like to emphasize that the calcium-losing effect of protein on the human body is not an area of controversy in scientific circles. The many studies performed during the past 55 years consistently show that the most important dietary change that we can make if we want to create positive calcium balance that will keep our bones solid is to decrease the amount of proteins we eat each day. The important change is not to increase the amount of calcium we take in."

He cites five different studies by five different research teams studying the effect of low- and

"I would counsel those who are not greatly troubled by postmenopausal symptoms, and who wish to protect themselves from the problems of osteoporosis and heart disease, to seek protection through improved nutrition (a low-fat, low-protein, high-fiber diet) and not through pills, tablets, or skin patches. It is unlikely that good health will come from a medicine bottle. If that were the case, how would we explain the striking lack of heart disease, osteoporosis, and cancer in areas of the world where these medications are not available? This observation deserves some additional comment. If you were to map out parts of the world where women suffer most from osteoporosis, you would color in the United States, Canada, the United Kingdom, and Europe. These are the very parts of the world where the most estrogens, progestins, calcium pills, and milk are used. The parts of the world without a serious osteoporosis problem are the very countries where there is virtually no estrogen, progestins, calcium pills, or milk. These countries include China, rural South America, and Africa. This irrefutable observation must be satisfactorily explained by advocates of dairy products, as well as estrogen and calcium supplementation."

—*Dr. Robert M. Kradjian,*
Save Yourself from Breast Cancer

high-protein diets on calcium balance. Each study found the same connection: The more protein that is ingested, the more calcium is lost, even if the dietary calcium is as high as 1,400 mg per day!

And, by the way, those new (or perhaps I should say resurrected) high-protein, low-carbohydrate weight-loss diets are dangerous for your bones. They force your body to use an inferior source of fuel: fat metabolites called ketones, which cause your kidneys to go into overdrive because they are toxic and the body needs to flush them out of the system. This is why someone in a hyperketonic state has bad breath. Water is drained from the tissues for this purpose, causing dehydration and strain on the kidneys. You can lose an impressive amount of weight quickly, but it's mostly water, and you lose some bone and muscle as well (more about this in the exercise section). You can become weak and dizzy, and your heart may race. As soon as you eat a normal diet, the water supply is restored, you feel better, your breath smells sweet again, and your weight returns.

Many insulin-resistant or carbohydrate-sensitive people go on this type of high-protein diet, mistakenly believing that the body treats all carbohydrates the same. A high-carbohydrate, low-fat diet made up of *complex* carbohydrates—whole grains, vegetables, fruits, and legumes— does not have the same effect on the body as a high-carbohydrate, low-fat diet made up of fat-free convenience foods. One study—see page 41 for more detail—showed that a low-fat convenience-food diet caused levels of triglycerides (a special molecule the body uses to transport fat in the blood) to go *up* 30 percent, and a plant-food diet with the same amount of calories, fat, saturated fat, carbohydrate, protein, and sugar caused triglycerides to go *down* 25 percent! With the plant-food diet, the sugar was almost all from fruit, and the carbohydrates contained the natural fiber and other nutrients missing from the processed convenience food. As the study director, Christopher Gardner of Stanford University, said, "You can't just talk about nutrients like fat and carbohydrates anymore. You have to talk about foods."

Soy to the rescue

So where does soy come in? Isn't soy a high-protein food? Yes, it is the highest-protein plant food. But it is comparatively lower in protein than meat and other animal products. A ½ cup serving of firm tofu has 13 g of protein, compared to an average hamburger, chicken drumstick, or piece of cod, all of which contain about 25 g of protein.

...and the Advisability of Calcium Supplementation

After careful research, I do not believe that calcium supplements are necessary or even advisable. It is easy to get enough calcium, even from a strictly plant-derived diet (see "Good Nondairy Sources of Calcium," pages 34-35, and menus on pages 28-29). Calcium needs to be balanced with magnesium and many other nutrients, so it is far better to get it in your food than in supplements. You'd be better off using the time spent worrying about calcium intake to participate in weight-bearing activities, quit smoking, get enough vitamin D, and plan healthful, well-balanced, animal-protein-free meals!

Our bodies absorb the calcium found in foods at varying rates. Low-oxalate vegetables such as kale, broccoli, turnip and mustard greens, and collards have a higher rate of calcium absorbability than milk products, for instance. Eating a varied diet, taking advantage of the rich array of plant foods available to us, will satisfy your calcium needs.

Furthermore, it seems that all protein is not created equal when it comes to affecting calcium balance. Dr. Neal Breslau of the University of Texas Health Science Center tested the effects of different types of protein on calcium balance in 1988. Subjects ate diets containing the same amounts of protein and calcium, but the protein was in three different forms: meat and cheese in one group; soyfoods, cheese, and eggs in another group; and soyfoods only in the third group. The meat-and-cheese group excreted 50 percent more calcium from their bodies than the soyfoods-only group. The soy, egg, and cheese group fell somewhere in the middle.

These results echoed those of some animal experiments performed the same year by Dr. Dike Kalu, also of the University of Texas Health Science Center, who compared the effects of soy protein with those of milk protein on bone health and kidney function of rats. The rats consuming soy protein showed a delay in the onset of age-related increase in bone loss, and their total amount of bone loss was significantly less. This study suggests that consuming soyfoods from an early age may help prevent osteoporosis.

No one is certain just why soy protein seems to affect calcium balance in a way that's different from animal protein. It may be that soy protein is low in amino acids that contain sulfur, which causes production of the chemical sulfate in the urine. Sulfate keeps calcium from being reabsorbed into the blood by the kidneys and, instead, filters calcium out of the body through the urine. Thus, low levels of sulfur in soy protein help protect your bones.

Another way that soy may help bone density is with the isoflavone daidzein, which is found primarily in soy products. This anticarcinogenic isoflavone also may have some bone-developing qualities. Recent studies at the University of North Carolina have found that even in low doses, genistein, an isoflavone found only in soy, prevents bone loss almost as well as estrogen therapy. This may be due to genistein's weak estrogenic properties. It's possible that the plant estrogens in soy may bind to estrogen receptors in the body, including the ones in our bone cells. This may help maintain bone tissue in much the same way as our own naturally produced estrogen.

Because plant estrogens are weaker, you need to eat at least 90 mg of isoflavones in soyfoods per day in order to see the effects, according to a study done at the University of Illinois. Some experts say that three to eight servings of soyfoods a day, with an of average 40 mg isoflavones per serving or 120 to 360 mg per day, is a bone-protective dose of soy foods. Three servings of soyfoods might include half a cup of tofu in a stir-fry for dinner and two cups of soymilk (for instance, on breakfast cereal; in a shake, cocoa, tea, or coffee; and used in cooking and baking throughout the day), which adds up to about 120 mg of isoflavones. So you see that it's not at all difficult to get the basic amount in food.

You also can add little bits of soy to meals throughout the day. For instance, ½ cup of reconstituted textured soy protein in canned vegetarian chili for lunch, ¼ cup of roasted soynuts for a snack, ¼ cup soy protein isolate powder mixed with a serving of soymilk in a shake or a cup of cocoa, ½ cup of green soybeans in a vegetable salad, a few table-spoons of tofu sour cream on a potato, and a little soy flour in your bread will quickly increase the amount you take in to the optimum eight servings.

Current studies are examining whether or not isoflavones work when ingested alone as a supplement in pill or powder form, as opposed to being eaten in their natural form along with the soy protein in food. For the time being, it seems that the safer and more reliable route—more enjoyable, and cheaper too—is to get your isoflavones in soyfoods, not from supplements. It may turn out that you can overdose on isoflavones taken as supplements, but it's highly unlikely that you could overdose on them through food, unless you ate nothing but soyfoods. Research may also discover that there are components in soyfoods that we don't know about yet that help the isoflavones do their work.

Soybeans are rich not only in protein, isoflavones, and calcium but also in magnesium, which regulates active calcium transport throughout the body, activates vitamin D, and helps the functions of bone-related hor-mones parathyroid and calcitonin. The trace element boron is also found in soybeans, while meat and fish are poor sources. One study found that boron supplementation markedly reduced urinary excretion of calcium and magnesium and also raised the level of an estrogen called estradiol-17 beta. Because this type of estrogen has the greatest impact on the body, boron may be an important nutritional factor in preventing osteoporosis.

The exercise factor: how you can regain lost bone density and stop middle-age spread

Whenever osteoporosis is addressed in the mainstream press, calcium intake—or, usually, *dairy* intake—is front and center, with little or no mention of the factors that interfere with its absorption or hasten its loss from the body. The importance of vitamin D and other nutrients also may be mentioned, along with other risk factors such as smoking and heavy drinking. For menopausal women, hormone replacement therapy usually is highly recommended. In the mainstream media, exercise typically is only mentioned in passing.

However, innumerable studies show that high calcium intake does not necessarily prevent bone loss, and it *cannot* build bone after the growing period—but exercise can! I have never been an athletic person, but the new research on exercise and bone health has motivated me to keep up a daily exercise program that I will never give up. I find it so empowering that there is something we can do on our own, in our own homes without spending lots of money, that can heal ourselves and prevent further degeneration, and that has many other physical and psychological benefits.

Our bodies were made to move and to work hard. Weight-bearing exercise stimulates the bone-rebuilding process and promotes maximum bone density. To quote a succinct explanation of the process from Dr. Joyce Vedral's book *Definition* (Warner Books, 1995): "Bone is a living tissue composed of calcium phosphate and the protein collagen. There are hundreds of concentric rings inside the bone (these are called haversian canals). When significant force is exerted upon a bone to which a working muscle is attached, an increased blood flow surges through the bone with nutrients. Eventually the bone builds more cells and thickens. In addition, the stress upon the bone caused by lifting weights causes an electrical charge to shoot through the haversian canals and to further stimulate the cells of the bone. In summary, it is the combination of the increased blood flow and the stimulating electrical charge that causes the bones to thicken."

But you must exercise the whole body. Running or walking will benefit your leg bones, but you also must do upper body weight training to build up the bones in your arms and torso.

Until very recently, the conventional wisdom was that you achieved your peak bone mass between the ages of 25 and 35, and after that, all you could hope for was to slow down the inevitable loss in bone density. And certainly it has been shown that, in sedentary people, bone mass and bone calcium deplete rapidly. A totally sedentary lifestyle, as in older adults sitting listlessly in front of televisions in nursing homes, will undermine calcium metabolism to the point that no amount of calcium supplementation or other nutritional therapy can help.

But many recent studies show that exercise can turn back the clock and that, indeed, weight-bearing exercise is the only known way to build bone density after we have stopped growing. A study at the University of Wisconsin by Dr. Everett Smith demonstrated that even 90-year-olds can regain muscle tone and increase bone density in their legs and hips by marching in place while holding onto a support. Lifting small hand weights could do the same for the upper body.

Dr. William Evans at Tufts University found that men and women ages 87 to 96 could increase the strength in their thighs by an average of 175 percent in just eight weeks of strength training.

Dr. Miriam E. Nelson has been studying the health benefits of strength training at Tufts University for more than ten years. Her research, published in the *Journal of the American Medical Association*, shows that women get stronger, build bone, improve balance and flexibility, and increase their energy through a moderate program of weight training.

So, if you don't already exercise, start now. You don't have to become a jogger; just get out and walk briskly every day, or do some energetic dancing, if that's more your style. (I belly dance and walk.) Other aerobic activities include using a treadmill or a stair stepper, jogging or jumping rope on a minitrampoline, doing step aerobics, in-line skating, and hiking.

And, just as important, start a moderate weight-training program. You can join a gym and use its equipment or simply use hand weights in your own home, which is what I do. (See the bibliography on pages 178-181 for some good instructional books.) Some studies have shown that people who work out at home keep it up longer and more consistently than do people who go to gyms. Working out on resistance machines or elastic resistance bands, such as Jump Stretch Inc. bands, is great for people who have difficulty handling weights, and rowing machines or exercise bikes ("spinning") with increased resistance on the flywheel are also good ways to strengthen bones. Just make sure to do a variety of activities that use different muscles, and include stretching in your program.

If you need to lose weight, a combination of aerobic activity and weight training will take off pounds. I lost twenty pounds and more than eighteen inches in less than a year, with no change in diet. This is a much more healthful way to lose weight than dieting. You actually lose muscle and bone when you diet, even "sensibly." According to registered dietician Debra Waterhouse, author of *Outsmarting the Midlife Fat Cell* (Hyperion, 1998), dieting during menopause is even more detrimental than dieting at any other time of your life, because you lose muscle faster and your fat cells store fat more easily if you lower your calorie level. Fat cells, which store estrogen, become larger and even more efficient at using calories as your ovaries produce less estrogen, particularly the fat cells around your middle body—this is middle-aged spread. Soyfoods, which can balance your estrogenic levels, may actually help you stay slim, according to registered dietician Elizabeth Somer, author of *Age-Proof Your Body* (William Morrow, 1998).

No matter how much protein and calcium you ingest, 20 to 30 percent of the weight lost through dieting is water, bone, muscle, and other lean tissue. The faster you lose, the larger the proportion of your loss is *not* fat. A 1994 study at Queens Medical Centre in Nottingham, England, found that premenopausal women who dieted moderately and lost an average of 7.5 lbs. in three months lost 1 percent bone mass as well. Premenopausal women normally lose no more than 0.5 percent per year. Strength training can prevent this by replacing fat with muscle. A pound of muscle takes up five to seven times less space than a pound of fat, so you will look slimmer even if you stay the same weight.

Many nutritionists believe that with even moderate dieting—eating about 1,200 calories a day—women cannot ingest enough food to give them adequate nutrition and that in order to consume enough essential nutrients, women need at least 1,800 calories per day of a balanced, varied diet.

A weight-loss study at Baylor College in Houston, Texas, recently compared the success rate of three groups: a diet-only group (1,200 calories per day); a diet-and-exercise group (same diet plus some form of exercise three to five times per week); and an exercise-only group. In one year the diet-only group shed an average of 15 pounds, the diet-and-exercise group lost an average of 20 pounds, and the exercise-only group lost an average of just six pounds. However, by the second year of the study the diet-only group had regained an average of 13 pounds, and the combination group had regained an average of 15 pounds. But the exercise-only group had regained an average of only a pound. These subjects were actually better off than the diet-only group by an average of three pounds; they ended up with the same actual loss as the diet-and-exercise group, but without dieting!

Ken Goodrick, one of the study leaders, explains that dieting is just too difficult for most people to stay with it. Exercise offers a slower loss but many other benefits, including increased motivation to eat a balanced, healthful diet.

So the sooner you start exercising, the better. Make it a habit as early in life as you can. Younger women benefit by increasing their peak bone mass; they find exercise a mood enhancer and immune system booster, and it can be helpful for PMS. But it's never too late. A one-year study at the University of Missouri showed that previously sedentary postmenopausal women who did both low- and high-impact exercise for as little as three twenty-minute sessions a week were able to

A day's supply of calcium from food alone

This vegan menu, from Food for Life, *by Dr. Neal Barnard (Harmony Books, 1993), provides more than 800 mg of calcium. It is a very simple menu—no snacks or even soy, except what might be used in the pancakes or cornbread—with moderate portions of food:*

Breakfast: 3 medium pancakes and 1 orange (196 mg)

Lunch: 1⅓ cup Campbell's Lentil Soup; 1 cup romaine lettuce with ½ tomato; 1 English muffin (170 mg)

Dinner: 1 cup vegetarian baked beans; 1 cup cooked broccoli; 2 ounces cornbread (439 mg)

Total for the day: 805 mg calcium

maintain their spinal bone density. Another study by researchers at Family Health International in Durham, North Carolina, found that women between the ages of 40 and 54 who were physically active had significantly higher bone density in the spine and arms than a comparable group of sedentary women.

My inspiration is Dr. Ruth Heidrich of Hawaii. Dr. Heidrich endured a double mastectomy in her late 50s and did not know if she had long to live. She embarked on a very low-fat vegan diet and a challenging exercise program, as much for her mental health as for her physical health. Now in her 60s, she has been cancer-free for many years. She is a veteran of the Ironman triathalons and holds multiple age-group records in Hawaii for races of every distance. She has written two books and travels around the world telling her story.

Amazingly, she has increased her bone density since age 50. Her bone density at 60 was higher than the average peak bone mass for a 30-year-old woman. She has been on a vegan diet—that means no dairy products—for several years, and has never taken estrogen or calcium. She credits this amazing achievement to exercise.

Another of my "mentors" is Dr. Joyce Vedral, whose books on weight training inspired me (and my husband) to start a home weight program that we intend to continue for life. She is in her 50s, a small woman, and she has also increased her bone density to almost double the density of the average woman of her age—her bones are more dense than even an in-shape 25-year-old! And she didn't touch a weight until she was in her 40s.

Here's another menu that I made up. It contains twice as much calcium—again, only from plant foods—as well as about 3½ servings of soy:

Breakfast: 1 cup hot fortified flavored soymilk and two 7-inch waffles (made with baking powder) (658 mg)

Lunch: vegetarian chili made with 1 cup cooked pinto beans and ⅓ cup reconstituted textured soy protein; 2 corn tortillas; 1 cup cooked kale (570 mg)

Snack: a shake made from the juice of one orange, ½ ounce soy protein isolate powder, 2½ ounces of silken tofu, and half a banana (160 mg)

Dinner: pasta e fagiole made from ½ cup cooked chick-peas, a carrot, and 1 cup cooked macaroni; 1 cup cooked broccoli; 1 slice bread (290)

Total for the day: 1,678

So, as you can see, it's easy to get enough calcium from foods, as long as you aren't just eating convenience foods.

These examples of increased bone density in older women are in stark contrast to much of the information that you will read. Most "experts" will tell you that *everyone* loses some bone mass "in the later years." While it is true that the more dense your bones are between the ages of 25 and 35 (peak bone mass), the less chance you have of developing osteoporosis later in life, you have a good chance of not only halting bone loss but actually increasing it by following the nutritional and lifestyle advice just discussed—and, most importantly, by exercising vigorously and regularly throughout life.

Other ways to protect your bones naturally

Besides eating less protein overall, using soy protein instead of animal protein (including dairy products), and eating a reasonable amount of calcium-rich plant foods (see "Good Nondairy Sources of Calcium," pages 34-35), and, of course, exercising, what else can you do to protect your bones?

✓ Take your vitamin D. Vitamin D is crucial because it regulates the metabolism of calcium and phosphorus. Yet most of us have been lulled into complacency about this vitamin because it has been added to dairy products. (It does not occur naturally in them.) Fifteen minutes of daily sun exposure to the face and arms (added up during the normal course of a day—you don't have to sunbathe) is enough to produce sufficient vitamin D supplies from a form of the vitamin produced in our livers and present on the skin. (People over 50 need slightly longer, because skin becomes less effective at absorbing vitamin D as we age. How much longer is a matter of variables, such as skin color, where one lives, etc.) But many people do not get this sort of exposure anymore due to our justifiable fear of skin cancer or the use of sunscreens, which, if they are applied faithfully and have a sun protection factor (SPF) of 8 or more, have been shown to interfere with vitamin D production.

In addition, people who live in cooler climates (for North Americans, this means north of Boston, Chicago, or Oregon, for example) have consistently lower blood levels of vitamin D than those living in more tropical climates. If vitamin D status is adequate, it appears that the body can absorb calcium more efficiently when calcium intake is low, but this may not compensate entirely for very low calcium intake during childhood, so make sure that your children eat calcium-rich plant foods *and* get their vitamin D. I take 400 mg of a plant-based vitamin D_2 tablet daily from October to April. Do not take more than 800 mg a day, as excessive amounts of vitamin D may cause more rapid calcium loss, and megadoses may create heart and kidney problems. During the sunny months (but not during the extreme heat of the day), I make sure to get about twenty minutes of sun exposure several times a week before I apply a sunscreen.

✓ Quit smoking or, better yet, never start. The chemically exposed ovaries of smoking women produce less estrogen, so they usually have a lower bone density *before* they start menopause. After menopause, smokers lose bone mass at a faster rate than nonsmokers.

✓ Cut down on caffeine consumption because it is thought to increase calcium excretion through the kidneys. This does not appear to be a serious problem with younger women unless they are heavy coffee consumers, but in postmenopausal women as little as two cups a day has been found to accelerate bone loss in those whose calcium intake is low.

✓ Excessive amounts of sodium in the diet seem to interfere with calcium absorption as well. This doesn't mean that you have to ban salt from your diet. You're already ahead of the game if you follow a vegan diet because it is estimated that 75 percent of the sodium in the North American diet comes from cheese and packaged foods, which you probably seldom eat. Milk and meat are both naturally high in sodium, and salt is added to cheese. If you go easy on pickled foods, salted nuts, chips, popcorn, and pretzels, as well as follow a vegan diet with few packaged foods, you can use soy sauce and miso and salt your food moderately.

✓ Too much phosphorous in the diet causes the body to excrete calcium in the feces. This is of particular interest to young women who may have low calcium intake to start with, then also drink a lot of phosphorous-laden soft drinks and eat meat, which is also high in phosphorous.

✓ Heavy drinking and alcoholism both reduce intestinal absorption and kidney excretion of calcium and other minerals. Intake of aluminum, from baking powders, antacids, and cooking pots, may also cause calcium excretion. Glucocorticoid therapy and other steroid-type drugs result in bone loss too.

✓ On the other hand, various nutrients in the diet boost calcium metabolism, calcium absorption, and bone formation: Vitamin K, vitamin C, vitamin B$_6$, folic acid, manganese, zinc, copper, silicon, and strontium are all important. Fortunately for vegetarians, these nutrients are found in dark leafy greens, fruits, whole grains, nuts and seeds, legumes, nutritional yeast, and fresh vegetables.

✓ Dr. Jerilynn Prior, professor of endocrinology at the University of British Columbia, has conducted numerous studies on the effects of stress and found an overall increased risk of osteoporosis in women who were stressed-out, too thin, overly concerned with their weight, and doing physical training that was too rigorous for their level of ability. A study in the *New England Journal of Medicine* showed that women who suffered from major depression, requiring therapy and antidepressants, had a lower bone density. Women who severely restrict calories probably have increased levels of the stress hormone cortisol, which causes calcium to be leached from the bones.

High-risk women

Your doctor or women's health clinic can tell you about new and inexpensive ways to test your bone density, such as heel ultrasound, which uses no radiation, takes only minutes, and costs just a few dollars to perform. Whatever your age, you should have this done so that you know whether you are at risk or not. The new inexpensive testing methods do not test bone density at the spine and hip, and may miss 20 to 30 percent of women with low bone density in these sites. So, if your test comes out normal (+1 to -1), but you are menopausal, have other significant risk factors (see "High Risk Factors for Osteoporosis," facing page), have broken a bone from a modest trauma, or are five to ten years past menopause, you may wish to ask your doctor for a DEXA test, which is not so readily available and is more expensive.

If you are in the high-risk group for osteoporosis and you have tried all of the above-mentioned advice, but your bone density is *still* threatened, *first and foremost*, get some professional advice about designing a more vigorous strength training and exercise program.

What about the new designer estrogens, or SERMs (Selective Estrogen Receptor Modulators), such as Raloxifene? According to Ethel Siris, an osteoporosis expert at Columbia-Presbyterian Hospital in New York City, Raloxifene is suitable only for postmenopausal women who aren't already taking estrogen and who don't already have osteoporosis. She feels that it is safe for the uterus and breasts, but it can still cause blood clots in the legs. Preliminary research also shows it has only a small benefit on cholesterol levels. I believe that if you follow all of the diet, exercise, and other lifestyle recommendations I have outlined, using Raloxifene as well would be expensive and probably redundant, and it is still not without risk.

Drugs like Fosomax, based on alendironate, a nonhormonal bone builder, are now often prescribed for older women with fragile bones, but Fosomax can cost more than $60 a month, which can put a severe strain on the budget of any woman on a senior's small fixed income. Even worse, women should know that it is a substance foreign to the human body and the bone that it makes is not exactly the same as normal human bone—it's more brittle. There have been no long-term studies for this drug, and *The New England Journal of Medicine* cited a 1996 study that called attention to an alarming number of women who suffered serious damage to their esophagi. If you don't drink enough water with the drug, complications can result. The drug company now recommends that patients remain sitting or standing for at least a half an hour after taking Fosomax and that they do not lie down immediately after. This drug is just too risky, in my opinion.

High Risk Factors for Osteoporosis

You're at increased risk of developing osteoporosis if you are:

Menopausal

Caucasian

Fair-skinned, with light hair and eyes

Under 5'2"

Thin and small-boned

Under stress

A smoker

A heavy drinker

A meat-eater

Sedentary with poor muscle tone

On thyroid or steroid medication

Having irregular periods and a history of eating disorders and/or extreme dieting

---

Good Nondairy Sources of Calcium

Several brands of soymilk and orange juice are fortified with calcium, vitamin D, and other nutrients. Check the labels for more information. Some ready-to-eat cold breakfast cereals are also fortified with calcium.

Nuts, such as almonds, and seeds, such as sesame, also provide calcium, but they are so high in fat that I would not depend on them as a regular source of calcium, so I have not listed them here. I also have not listed high-oxalate foods such as spinach, chard, beets, beet greens, parsley, and rhubarb. Although these are high in calcium, the oxalates prevent much of it from being available to the body. There is no need to avoid these foods, since they are high in other nutrients, but don't depend on them for calcium.

753 mg	3 ounces pressed or extra-firm tofu curdled with nigari and calcium sulphate
683 mg	3 ounces firm tofu curdled with calcium sulphate
377 mg	3 ounces pressed or extra-firm tofu made with nigari
357 mg	1 cup cooked collard greens
350 mg	3 ounces medium-firm tofu curdled with calcium suphate
280 mg	2 tablespoons blackstrap molasses
258 mg	½ cup (4 ounces) firm tofu made with nigari
252 mg	1 cup cooked turnip greens
232 mg	½ cup dry-roasted soybeans
206 mg	1 cup cooked kale
205 mg	3 ounces firm tofu curdled with magnesium chloride
200-300 mg	1 teaspoon baking powder

196 mg	2 corn tortillas or 16 baked tortilla chips
193 mg	1 cup cooked mustard greens
179 mg	7-inch waffle (made with baking powder),
176 mg	1 cup cooked okra
78 mg	1 cup cooked broccoli
158 mg	1 cup cooked bok choy
145 mg	3 ounces boiled green soybeans
115 mg	½ cup masa harina (the special corn flour used to make tortillas)
108 mg	1 cup baked acorn squash
125 mg	½ (12.3-ounce) package silken tofu
105 mg	3 ounces medium-firm tofu curdled with magnesium chloride
102 mg	1 ounce soy protein isolate powder
100 mg	4 ounces soy tempeh
100 mg	1 cup cooked chick-peas, white beans, or pinto beans
88 mg	½ cup cooked dried soybeans
83 mg	½ cup carrot juice
68 mg	¼ cup dry textured soy protein (½ cup reconstituted)
62 mg	1 cup cooked green beans
56 mg	1 cup cooked potato
49 mg	½ cup okara (soybean pulp from making tofu or soymilk),
45 mg	1 tablespoon naturally fermented soy sauce

Chapter 3

Preventing the number one killer of women (as well as men)—heart disease

When women are asked what disease they fear most, the majority will say breast cancer. What most women don't know is that *they are six times more likely to die of a heart attack than of breast cancer*. Heart disease is, in fact, the number one killer of North American women. It kills more women every year than all cancers, lung disease, pneumonia, diabetes, accidents, and AIDS *combined*. Sixty percent of the sudden deaths of North American women are attributed to heart attacks, most without prior warning.

Women are becoming more informed about osteoporosis and breast cancer, but they are still woefully ignorant about heart disease, its prevalence, and the differences in symptoms, testing, and treatments for men and women. Unfortunately, many doctors are uninformed about these differences too, and they think of heart disease as a men's problem. Medical staff who are not educated about the symptoms many women display when having a heart attack may misdiagnose a heart attack as the flu or even just fatigue. For this reason, *women are twice as likely to die within a few weeks after their first heart attack than men*. In fact, as of 1990, more American women died of heart attacks than men.

> ### Some unfortunate facts about North American women
>
> *25 percent smoke*
>
> *35 percent are overweight*
>
> *40 percent over age 50 have high cholesterol levels*
>
> *60 percent are sedentary*
>
> *75 percent over 65 have high cholesterol levels*
>
> *All of these are risk factors for heart disease. Women who undergo angioplasty and coronary bypass surgery are twice as likely to die from complications as men.*

Age is a major risk factor for heart disease in women. Of the approximately 247,000 fatal female heart attacks that occur in the United States every year, only about 6,500 occur in women under the age of 65. Estrogen is believed to protect the heart and blood vessels from the effects of heart disease, so menopausal women should be aware of other ways to protect themselves from this killer. One of these protective factors is soy.

In *The Simple Soybean and Your Health*, Dr. Mark Messina and Virginia Messina write: "Scientists have known for close to a hundred years that the protein you eat helps to determine your chances of getting a heart attack. Around the turn of the century, it was reported that animal protein such as meat, eggs, and milk induces atherosclerosis. And more than a quarter century ago, studies showed, rather dramatically, that plant proteins lower cholesterol levels. In fact, some of the now-classic studies comparing heart-disease rates and saturated-fat intakes of different countries actually suggested that animal protein was one important reason for differences in these rates."

Some of the first human studies on soy protein and its effect on blood cholesterol levels took place in the 1960s. About ten years later, Italian scientists at the University of Milan found that soy protein lowered high cholesterol levels by 14 percent in two weeks, and 21 percent in three weeks. Since then, numerous studies have had similar results. Dr. Kenneth Carrol of the University of Western Ontario evaluated the results of 40 such studies on soy protein and came to a similar conclusion: Soy protein was most effective in people who had high cholesterol levels, the results had nothing to do with fat or cholesterol in the diet, and, most important, it was the LDL, or "bad" cholesterol, that was lowered. Other studies show that soy protein also raises HDL levels, or "good" cholesterol.

There have been several studies showing that simply adding as little as 20 grams of soy protein to a person's normal diet each day, with no other changes, can lower cholesterol levels by 10 percent or more. Replacing animal protein in the diet with soy protein and lowering fat levels can decrease the levels even more dramatically. This dietary route, along with exercise, stress reduction, and not smoking, is a viable alternative to the expense and potentially dangerous side effects of cholesterol-lowering drugs.

No one is quite sure just *how* soy protein works—just that it does. One theory is that the low levels of the amino acid lysine in soy and other vegetable proteins is responsible; animal protein has a high lysine content. Lysine raises insulin levels, thereby speeding up the production of cholesterol by the body. This may explain why a so-called prudent diet, which contains liberal amounts of lean meats and low-fat dairy products, does not lower cholesterol levels as dramatically as a low-fat vegetarian diet does.

Australian researchers illustrated this quite clearly in a study of subjects who were all on diets containing 30 percent of calories from fat. One group ate the "prudent" diet containing lean meat. The other group ate the same amount of fat but plant proteins only. The plant-protein diet was twice as effective as the prudent diet at lowering cholesterol levels.

There are other components of soy that may also help to lower cholesterol levels. One of these is fiber. Do you remember oat bran? For a few years manufacturers were throwing oat bran into every imaginable food product. Oat bran does produce a modest decrease in cholesterol levels because it contains soluble fiber, or fiber that is soluble in water. Soluble fiber moves through the small intestine and seems to interfere with the absorption of cholesterol. About 30 percent of the fiber in soybeans is soluble; other fruits, vegetables, grains, and legumes also contain soluble fiber. Soybeans can be part of a healthful plant-based diet, which naturally contains high levels of fiber. Because some soyfoods, such as tofu, contain little fiber, choose whole, cooked soybeans, textured soy protein, roasted soynuts, and green soybeans for their fiber content.

The antioxidants in soy may play a protective role in preventing heart disease. Many scientists believe that damage to the arterial wall occurs due to oxidation of LDL, caused by free radicals, unstable oxygen molecules. Japanese researchers found that soy protein decreased the production of oxidized and deformed LDL and concluded that this might be useful in preventing hardening of the arteries.

The isoflavone genistein, of which we have heard much, is believed to inhibit the action of enzymes that promote cell growth and migration. Some researchers speculate that genistein thus prevents the growth of cells that form plaque deposits in the arteries, in much the same way that it seems to prevent the growth of tumors. This is being studied at the University of Washington, along with a theory that genistein inhibits cell stickiness. Josiah Wilcox and Barbara Blumenthal of the Division of Hematology and Oncology at Emory University Medical School believe that genistein may prevent the progression of hardening and clogging of the arteries and blood vessels by inhibiting the formation of the enzyme thrombin, which helps blood clot. Thrombin appears at the sites of cell lining injuries in the blood vessels and the clot formation they promote leads to hard, fatty lumps or atherosclerotic plaques. Susan Potter, principal investigator in the soy-cholesterol studies at the University of Illinois, is looking at the effects of soy protein and soy isoflavones in relation to cardiovascular disease and osteoporosis in women. Preliminary findings show that soy protein apparently lowered the subject women's blood cholesterol by 10 to 25 percent.

Saponins, which are compounds derived from sugars that occur in many plants (particularly legumes), resemble cholesterol in their chemical makeup. They also are thought to lower cholesterol either by blocking cholesterol absorption or by causing more cholesterol to be excreted from the body. It was noted in an article on saponins appearing in a 1981 issue of Food Chemistry that the increase in heart disease in Western societies coincided with a decrease in the consumption of saponin-rich legumes.

Those soy estrogens that we hear so much about may also lower cholesterol levels by exerting an estrogenic effect on the body. Estrogen plays a big role in the way the body produces, handles, breaks down, and eliminates fats, which contribute to cholesterol levels. As we mentioned before, a woman's risk of developing heart disease rises sharply as her estrogen production drops.

There are many other components of soy that are being studied for their effects on heart disease: phytic acid, lecithin, essential fatty acids, magnesium, phytosterols, B vitamins . . . It is likely that a combination of all or many of these components is what makes soy such a heart-healthy food. In addition, substituting soy products for many high-calorie, high-fat meat and dairy products may help to prevent obesity in many people, and obesity can be a factor in heart disease and stroke.

A heart-healthy diet should include soy, but it should also be a plant-based diet that is low in fats and high in the complex carbohydrates (grains, fruits, vegetables, and legumes) that contain antioxidants. Soy does seem to have the most dramatic effects on people with high blood cholesterol levels, but it cannot cancel out other risk factors for heart disease.

What are these risk factors? Besides women in menopause, people with family histories of heart disease, stroke, and diabetes are considered at risk. If you are high risk, have your blood pressure checked regularly, and, if it's too high, exercise, limit alcohol, and eat a low-fat, plant-based diet. Losing as little as five or ten pounds can lower your blood pressure.

Get off the treadmill
Treadmill tests of heart health are not accurate for women. Ask for a stress echocardiogram test—it is accurate, sensitive, fairly quick, and involves no radioactive injections, as some tests do.

Have your cholesterol checked annually once you're over the age of 50, and use the same methods mentioned previously to keep your cholesterol levels healthy. *By the age of 55, high cholesterol threatens more women than men.* Unfortunately, younger women with low cholesterol may feel invincible and ignore healthy eating and exercise habits. Start good habits while you are young, and you may prevent serious problems as you age!

If you have *diabetes*, maintain a healthy weight, stay active, and reduce the fat in your diet. Many studies have shown that unprocessed soy (cooked dried whole soybeans, soy sprouts, soynuts, and green soybeans) may prove therapeutic in the treatment of diabetes. The addition of soy fiber to meals significantly reduced blood sugar and blood triglycerides in studies of obese diabetic patients.

What is a healthy level of cholesterol?

The official guidelines have recommended total cholesterol levels of below 200 mg/dl Between 200 and 239 generally is considered borderline high, but not worrisome unless you have established heart disease or two other risk factors. However, Dr. William Castelli, director of the famous Framingham heart study, tells us that 240 is the average cholesterol count of those who have suffered heart attacks! Dr. Castelli notes that most heart attacks occur in people with total cholesterol in the 200-240 range, but he has never seen a heart attack in anyone with a total cholesterol level of under 150 mg/dl He further tells us that data suggests that for each 1 percent rise in cholesterol, the risk of a heart attack increases by 2 to 3 percent.

Women are finally becoming the subject of cholesterol studies, and it appears that measuring the ratio of your total cholesterol to your HDL, or "good" cholesterol, is more accurate. According to the latest research, a ratio of less than 3.5 is desirable, between 3.5 and 6.9 constitutes moderate risk, and over 7.0 is dangerous. But while a ratio of 5.0 may be considered average risk, it means that you have a 50 percent chance of having a heart attack! By the way, long-term vegetarians have the lowest ratio of all groups—lower than marathon runners—with an average ratio of 2.8. And in two studies, one in the United States in 1985 and one in England in 1987, adding dairy, eggs, and fish to a vegan diet raised the ratio.

Women (and men) who smoke even lightly (one to four cigarettes a day) double their risk of heart disease. Smoking diminishes blood oxygen, which damages blood vessels, causes blood to thicken and blood platelets to become stickier, raises clotting factors and total cholesterol levels, and lowers the HDL ("good" cholesterol)—in effect, setting up an ideal climate for strokes and heart attacks.

High triglyceride levels are more powerful predictors of risk in women than in men. Triglyceride is another blood fat that plays a role in heart disease, but its role is not clearly understood. Furthermore, scientists do not agree on what is a safe level—they just agree that lower is better. Diabetes, kidney disease, and obesity can raise triglyceride levels, as can certain medications, including some diuretics, beta blockers, birth control pills, and other estrogen preparations. Losing weight—even as little as fifteen pounds—cutting back on sweets, drinking less alcohol, and exercising regularly can help control triglyceride levels.

In a small pilot study at Stanford University, researchers compared a low-fat "convenience food" diet with a low-fat, plant-food-based diet. They tested people with high cholesterol levels, rather than high triglyceride levels. Both diets had the same amounts of calories, fats, saturated fat, cholesterol, protein, and carbohydrates, but the convenience-food diet had things like fat-free cream cheese, fat-free cookies, low-fat bologna, and baked tortilla chips. The plant-food diet consisted of whole grains, salads, vegetables, and other whole foods. Both diets had about equal amounts of sugar, but in the plant-food diet it came mainly from fruit. The researchers reported that the difference in triglycerides between the two groups was "stunning." They went up 30 percent on the convenience-food diet and down 25 percent on the plant-food diet! This makes it doubtful that so-called insulin-resistant people need to go on high-protein diets and avoid high-complex-carbohydrate diets in order to keep their triglycerides from rising. A larger study is underway, and the lead researcher says that you can't just talk about nutrients like

Women have different heart attack symptoms than men

Women may have little or no chest pain. They may have shortness of breath and pain or weakness in the shoulder or arms, or all over the body. There may be nausea unrelieved by normal remedies. They may be vomiting. They may feel fatigued or totally wiped out, with a general sense of unwellness.

These symptoms may come and go, which signifies angina, a temporary lack of oxygen to the heart and a warning sign of future heart attacks. When these symptoms don't go away, and become worse as time passes, a heart attack could be happening, but it may be misdiagnosed as the flu. Because many people, including health professionals, assume that chest pain and tightness are the universal symptoms for heart attack, many women without chest pain are misdiagnosed. Women are twice as likely as men to die once they have a heart attack.

Don't delay. Call your doctor. Take an aspirin—taking one early in a heart attack has been shown to improve the rate of survival in both men and women. Go to the emergency room at the nearest hospital. Don't worry about being embarrassed if you really do have the flu. Be specific about symptoms and ask for a stress echocardiogram test.

carbohydrates and fats; you have to talk about specific foods that affect triglycerides.

Stress is another risk factor for heart disease. This has been known for many years. According to the famous Framingham heart study, when other risk factors are present, stress heightens their impact, increasing vulnerability. Also, when we experience stress, we may try to seek relief by drinking too much alcohol, smoking, or overeating, which are all further risk factors. If it is not possible to eliminate the stress from your life, remember that feelings of satisfaction and high levels of self-esteem seem to mitigate the stress, so seek activities and companions that foster these feelings. Seek relief and release through laughing (watch your favorite comedy), being with loved ones, pursuing satisfying hobbies, and engaging in vigorous exercise. When I have been in stressful periods of my life, I have found that walking, particularly near water, and dancing were very helpful to me. Many people are helped by learning to meditate, or pursuing such meditative activities as tai chi, yoga, and martial arts.

Depression and social isolation also are now considered risk factors and should be taken seriously. The recommendations for dealing with stress can also be helpful for depression. St. John's wort is an herb that many people have found helpful and nonaddictive for dealing with mild to moderate depression. A homeopathic practitioner also may be able to help. Try to build up your own personal social safety net of friends and family—healthy give-and-take relationships.

A *sedentary lifestyle* is nearly as dangerous as smoking and having high cholesterol, and is far more prevalent than both. It is the *MOST common modifiable risk factor*. Regular exercise lowers the resting pulse rate and blood pressure. It reduces total cholesterol and improves the ratio of "good" to "bad" cholesterol. It helps prevent diabetes and osteoporosis. It releases stress and tempers the craving for nicotine. It is also the only reliable way to control obesity, which is another risk factor.

Obesity appears to more than double the risk of heart attacks and, among women with coronary artery disease, 70 percent are significantly overweight. Obesity often goes hand in hand with other risk factors, such as high blood pressure, high cholesterol, high triglycerides, and diabetes, and often, as weight goes down, so do these risk factors. *But not necessarily*. I don't want to place too much emphasis on losing weight, or give the impression that being thin makes you immune to heart disease—it doesn't. I find that naturally thin people are often complacent about their heart health, not taking other risk factors such as lack of exercise, poor diet, or smoking into consideration, while otherwise very healthy, active overweight people are made to worry unnecessarily. If you are one of those people who will never be slim, but you exercise vigorously and regularly, eat a nutritious low-fat diet, don't smoke, and have your cholesterol and blood pressure checked regularly, keep doing what you are doing and don't be tempted to try harmful high-protein or extremely low-calorie weight-loss diets. (See Chapter 2 for more on weight loss.)

At any rate, it seems that it is not really your weight that counts, so much as where the pounds are situated on your body. It has been known since 1956 that apple-shaped women, who carry excess weight around their middles, rather than on their hips, thighs, and buttocks, are more vulnerable to high blood pressure, high cholesterol, and diabetes. This has been confirmed by many other studies since then, leading one researcher to suggest that heart disease should be compared in pear-shaped versus apple-shaped people, not men and women.

The potbelly, no-waistline, apple profile, as opposed to the fat-below-the-waist, pear shape contributes to changes in our insulin and fatty-acid production and predisposes us to the development of coronary artery disease. Abdominal obesity causes fatty acids and triglycerides to be poured into major veins from the abdominal fat cells and settle as plaque in our blood vessels.

A waist-to-hip ratio of greater than 0.8 indicates cardiac risk. To figure out your ratio, divide your waist measurement by your hip measurement. A low-fat, plant-based diet, with soy products taking the place of meat and dairy, and regular exercise, including weight training or resistance training, can help you lose weight. You may not ever be what you consider slim, but you will most likely reduce your waist-to-hip ratio, and become stronger and fitter in the process.

Chapter 4

Can soy prevent cancer?

One of the most publicized health benefits of soy is the possibility that it contains a number of cancer-fighting properties. It is more difficult to study the connection between soy and cancer prevention than soy and heart disease prevention, because there is a fairly reliable indicator, or biomarker, to measure in heart disease, namely, blood cholesterol. However, there are some chemicals, genes, fluids, and other substances in the body that are believed to predict development of cancers.

There are a number of studies being conducted at this time on volunteers at high risk of developing breast, prostate, or colon cancers with these biomarkers in mind. However, there are enough significant indicators from earlier studies and population statistics to make many experts recommend that we all add soy to our diets *now*, rather than wait the fifteen years or so that it may take to get the results of these studies.

One of the factors that sparked the interest of cancer researchers some years ago was the striking difference between mortality rates for breast cancer and prostate cancer in North America and Europe compared to Asian countries, such as China, Japan, the Republic of Korea, and Thailand. In the West, your chances of dying of breast or prostate cancer can be ten to twenty times higher than if you lived in one of these Asian countries.

Only a small number of cancers can be attributed to heredity. When Asians emigrate to Western countries, within a couple of generations their descendants catch right up to other Westerners in terms of cancer deaths. Even in Asia itself, as the diet has become more Westernized, there has been a slow but steady rise in mortality from all types of cancer.

Studies of Japanese men on traditional high-fiber, high-vegetable, low-fat diets show consistently that, though Japanese men get prostate cancer at the same rate as North American men, far fewer Japanese die from the disease, because the cancer does not grow or progress. When Japanese men move to North America and eat more Westernized diets, cancers are faster-growing.

Although it has not been clinically proven—an argument you will hear time and time again from dairy boards and meat producers—you don't have to be a rocket scientist to conclude that the Western high-fat, high-protein, low-fiber diet might have something to do with this discrepancy.

The seven countries with the highest rates of breast cancer (more than 20 deaths per 100,000 people per year) are countries where the average intake of fat is the highest (about 150 grams a day). The seven countries with the lowest rates of breast cancer (about 5 deaths per 100,000) occur in countries with the lowest intake of fats (less than 50 grams a day). Prostate cancer rates are very similar.

However, another major protective factor may be soy in the Asian diet. A major twenty-year study of 8,000 Japanese men in Hawaii found a direct correlation between tofu consumption and lower rates of prostate cancer. Those who consumed tofu once a week or less were three times as likely to get prostate cancer as those who ate it daily. Other factors were measured, *including fat intake*, and tofu consumption was deemed to be most protective.

Japan's average daily soy intake is 30 grams, whereas in the United States it is negligible. Japan's breast cancer death rate is 6 per 100,000 people, and the U. S. rate is 22 per 100,000. Japan's prostate cancer death rate is 4 per 100,000, and the U.S. rate is 16.

Cancer is believed to be a two-stage process: initiation, or exposure to a cancer-causing substance, and promotion, or stimulation by another substance that makes the first become active. There is considerable research going on today into substances that prevent the promotion stage and therefore halt or reverse cancer development. This is possible because ten years or more may pass between the time of tumor initiation and actual malignancy.

Soybeans contain several factors that may inhibit cancer growth, which may explain why the Japanese men in those studies got prostate cancer but succumbed to it far less often than did their Western counterparts.

Protease inhibitors are substances found in the reproductive parts of soybeans and other vegetables. Because they block the activity of an enzyme that aids the digestion of proteins, they were once thought to interfere with nutrition. The U.S. Dept. of Agriculture spent a lot of time and money trying to remove protease inhibitors from soybeans because they thought their removal would improve growth in children. However, it has been established that protease inhibitors are capable of neutralizing the effects of a large number of cancer-causing agents. Dr. Ann Kennedy, then of Harvard, now a leading researcher at the University of Pennsylvania School of Medicine, reported that even brief exposure of initiated and/or promoted cells to a particular protease inhibitor called BBI (derived from soybeans) not only prevented transformation of the cells into cancers, but also "reprogrammmed" the cells back to the "pre-initiation" stage.

In many laboratory studies, scientists have investigated protease inhibitors, especially BBI, and found that they inhibited cancers of the colon, lung, pancreas, mouth, esophagus, skin, and bladder. Evidently, protease inhibitors prevent the activation of specific genes that cause cancer, and they also protect against the damaging effects of free radicals and radiation.

There are other substances in soybeans and other plant foods that seem to have anticancer properties as well. *Polyphenols* have been reported to interfere with tumor promotion and to act as garbage collectors, disposing of cell-damaging mutagens and cancer-causing agents. *Phytates*, the plant storage form of the mineral phosphorus, abundant in soybeans, is a chelator, or a substance that binds with certain metals that may promote tumor growth and also acts as an antioxidant, preventing free radical damage. *Phytosterols* are related to cholesterols but are found only in plant foods and move straight through our intestines to our colons, protecting them against the harmful effects of bile acids and reducing the development of colon tumors. *Saponins* are antioxidants that protect against free radical damage and, in laboratory investigations, have been shown to prevent mutations that can lead to cancer.

All of these substances, and several others that are still being investigated, occur in many plant foods, which is one very good reason why you should eat a plant-based diet with a wide variety of vegetables, fruits, grains, and legumes. But soy contains them all, and more, which makes soy a valuable and potentially protective food.

Mark Messina, Ph.D., and Virginia Messina, in their wonderfully informative book *The Simple Soybean and Your Health*, point out the intriguing results of more than thirty different epidemiologic studies that have been conducted on many types of cancers and many varieties of soyfoods. Most of these studies were comparisons between people living in different parts of Asia, who had generally similar diets and lifestyles, including fat intake. It's more useful to compare these diets than Western and Asian diets, which have radically different average rates of fat consumption. The studies suggest that people who frequently consume soyfoods have lower cancer rates than those who consume soyfoods less often. Based on many of the studies, it seems that people who eat soyfoods daily have about half the risk of cancer as those who eat soyfoods only once or twice a week. For instance, a study in Singapore found that those women with the highest soyfood consumption had less than half the breast cancer risk of those who consumed soyfoods only rarely. A Japanese study showed that people who ate soy had only one-seventh the risk of rectal cancer of those who did not eat soy, and that eating soybeans and tofu lowered the colon cancer risk by 40 percent. In China, frequent consumers of soymilk had less than half the stomach cancer risk of those who did not drink it. Several studies in China, where smoking is more prevalent than in North America, found that lung cancer risk could be lowered by half with frequent consumption of tofu and other soyfoods.

One thing that makes soy truly unique as a protective food is that it is one of the few foods that contains significant amounts of plant estrogens or phytoestrogens called *isoflavones*. These plant compounds are converted during the normal digestive process into a form of very weak estrogen. Back in 1982, Dr. Kenneth Setchell, professor of Pediatrics at Children's Hospital and Medical Center in Cincinnati, identified a phytoestrogen called equol in the urine of people who eat soyfoods. Equol is structurally similar to the natural estrogen estradiol-17. Later, Dr. Herman Aldercreutz of the University of Helsinki found high levels of equol in the urine of Japanese men and women who ate a soy-rich traditional diet. He found low levels of equol in women who had breast cancer, as opposed to cancer-free women.

Scientists from several countries have found much higher levels of another isoflavone called *genistein* in the urine of people eating a traditional Japanese soy-rich diet than in those eating a typical Western diet. Genistein is a powerful anticarcinogen, *found only in soybeans*. It appears to inhibit enzymes that promote tumor growth. Test-tube experiments show that genistein can block the growth of prostate cancer cells and breast cancer cells. Also, genistein helps to promote something called differentiation in cancerous cells. To explain this simply, the human body has specialized cells—bone cells, heart cells, skin cells, etc.—that have unique properties. When cells become cancerous, they forget what they were designed to be and begin to look the same. These so-called undifferentiated cells are very resistant to cancer therapies.

Another isoflavone found in soy is *daidzein*. Studies show that this isoflavone can also inhibit the growth of cancer cells and promote cell differentiation.

Plant lignans are other phytoestrogens that occur widely in plant foods. Lignans are reported to have anticancer, antiviral, bactericidal, and fungistatic properties, and vegetarians have higher blood levels of them than do meat eaters.

Estrogens play a key role in the development of breast cancer. Among women who will eventually develop breast cancer, higher levels of active estrogen are present, apparently acting as a breast cancer promoter. For instance, estrogen increases cancer risk by binding to breast cells. Because isoflavones are so similar to human estrogen, they can attach to estrogen receptors, effectively blocking the human estrogen from latching on. But because isoflavones are much, much weaker than estrogen, they don't have the deadly effect that estrogens do. Tamoxifen, a breast-cancer drug, works in the same way.

Longer exposure to estrogen is a risk factor for breast cancer. Women who start to menstruate early and have a late menopause are at higher risk, because they have been exposed to potent estrogens for a longer period. Remaining childless and not breast-feeding are further risk factors, again because during pregnancy and round-the-clock breast-feeding (before periods return) there are less active forms of circulating estrogen than during menstruation.

One of the reasons that fat (and meat) in the diet may be a major factor in hormone-related cancers such as breast and prostate is that a high-fat diet promotes high estrogen levels. At the University of California School of Medicine in Los Angeles, David Heber placed women on a very low-fat diet—less than 10 percent of calories—for only three weeks. In that short time the women experienced a drop in serum estradiol levels (a form of estrogen) of an average of 50 percent; one dropped 80 percent! Another study in Boston measured blood hormone levels as well as urine excretion levels in vegetarian and meat-eating women. The vegetarian women had increased fecal excretion of estrogen, decreased levels of estrogen in the bile, and levels in the blood that were 11 to 20 percent lower than those in the meat-eating women. Many other studies, as well as epidemiologic research, point to a low-fat, low-meat diet as another way to lower the amount of estrogen exposure in a woman's lifetime.

A longer time between menstrual periods also reduces exposure to estrogen. Dr. Kenneth Setchell fed a group of women 60 grams of reconstituted textured soy protein daily for four weeks, and observed that the time between their menstrual cycles increased two to five days. Sixty grams of miso lengthened this by another day, though, admittedly, that is more miso than anyone would ever eat in a day.

(By the way, synthetic progestins have been linked to breast cancer. Natural progesterone produced by the body or derived from wild yams and soy, however, protects against breast cancer.)

Obesity after menopause is also considered a risk factor for cancer, because large amounts of estrogen can be made in the fatty tissue under the skin. This is another reason to become fit and as slim as your body is comfortable being (see Chapters 2 and 3).

Dr. Robert M. Kradjian, in his book *Save Yourself from Breast Cancer* (which I urge every woman and girl to read), paints a sad picture of the Western girl who, eating an estrogen-promoting, high-fat, high-protein diet, will start menstruating at about age 12, have only one or two children, and who will not breast-feed them for very long, if at all, thereby having a much longer exposure to potent estrogens than her sisters in less developed countries. About half of American girls exhibit breast or pubic hair development by age 9. In China, Japan, the Philippines, and Africa, where breast cancer rates are much lower, the average age of menarche (onset of menstruation) is 16 or 17, as it was in the United States 100 years ago. Breast-feeding is also prolonged, as it was 75 or more years ago in North America.

In men, estrogen also plays a part in prostate cancer. Estrogen is changed into androgen, a male hormone, and triggers the production of testosterone. Men with prostate cancer often have higher levels of testosterone than cancer-free men. The estrogen-blocking activities, as well as the tumor-inhibiting qualities, of soy isoflavones may therefore also play a part in preventing prostate cancer in men.

The cancer-protective claims for soy are called speculative by some, but the data is impressive. Soyfoods have clear benefits in protecting against heart disease and have been proven to have no negative side effects, so many scientists are advising us not to wait years for definitive studies, but to start reaping the benefits of the mighty soybean *now*.

And, of course, soy is only one part of a nutritious, protective diet. As I have mentioned before, it's not a magic bullet or a miracle food. A varied, complex-carbohydrate, high-fiber, low-fat, low-protein, plant-based diet with regular vigorous exercise is a most important component in a healthy life. As Dr. Robert M. Kradjian says (see page 21), it's unlikely that good health will come from a medicine bottle; we must seek protection from disease through improved nutrition. Adding soy to such a plan will only add more benefits, but this doesn't mean isolating this or that protective substance from the soybean and taking it in a supplemental form. We already know that we should get our antioxidants in the form of fresh fruits, vegetables, and legumes, because researchers haven't yet identified all the protective substances in food and aren't sure how they all work in concert with one another. Similarly, we aren't sure if the protective components of soybeans will work out of context. Isoflavones may not do their work if not accompanied by the soy protein, for instance. It is a lesson that we in the West have yet to learn—to trust the power of whole foods, rather than specific nutrients.

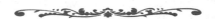

Chapter 5

A soy foods primer

From traditional Asian foods like tofu to recently developed Western products such as meat analogs and frozen nondairy desserts, there is now a vast array of soybean-based foods, known as *soyfoods*, to choose from. In this chapter, I'll briefly describe the different soyfoods that are called for in this book.

Many of these products are now available in large supermarkets, especially in areas with ethnically diverse populations. Otherwise, most of them are available in natural food stores or in Asian grocery stores. See the sources on pages 183-84 if you have trouble finding soyfoods in your area.

SOYBEANS

Whole dry soybeans are harvested when fully mature. Most varieties are yellow or beige in color, but there also are brown and black varieties available which are delicious. Whole soybeans are an excellent source of fiber, isoflavones, and protein; have the most calcium of any dry bean; and can be used in soups, casseroles, and bean dishes, as well as some dips. See pages 65-66 for instructions on cooking them.

When buying whole dried soybeans, look for beans that are mostly whole, with few split beans. They should be clean, with no dirt, stones, or foreign matter. They will keep for about a year if stored in a dry, cool area in a sealed container. Canned organic yellow and black soybeans are available in natural food stores.

SOY SPROUTS

Soy sprouts are nutritious and easy to grow at home from organic dried whole soybeans. The sprouts should not be eaten raw, but they need only brief stir-frying or steaming to make them edible—they should still be crunchy. The Chinese use soy sprouts as a base for vegetarian broth. Soy sprouts can be used in some recipes instead of green soybeans.

You may be able to find soy sprouts in Korean grocery stores, or try growing them yourself. Soy sprouts are grown the same as any large bean sprout, but they may take five to seven days to mature. The mature sprouts should be 1½ to 2½ inches long. Rinse them three times a day during growing. When the fully grown sprouts are placed in indirect sunlight for a few hours, they will turn green, which I find more appetizing. Before using, submerge in cold water and agitate; most of the hulls will then float to the top. Drain well and refrigerate in an airtight container until used.

SOY FLOUR _____

Soy flour is useful for adding soy's benefits to baked goods and can be found in natural food stores and some supermarkets. *Full-fat soy flour* is made from whole or hulled soybeans ground into a fine flour. It has the same composition as whole soybeans and so is extremely nutritious. It is usually sold in its raw (enzyme-active) form as opposed to the toasted form. The raw flour contains an enzyme, lipoxygenase, which serves as a dough conditioner, producing a moist, light bread that does not go stale quickly. Because of its high oil content, I keep full-fat soy flour in the freezer.

Defatted soy flour is made by grinding defatted soy flakes to a fine flour. It has a higher protein content than full-fat soy flour, as well as a higher isoflavone content. Some fat-soluble vitamins are removed, but most of the fiber, vitamins, minerals, and phytochemicals remain.

GREEN SOYBEANS _____

Green soybeans (edamamé, sweet beans) are picked at the peak of maturity, when they are still green and high in sucrose and chlorophyll. They have a color, texture, and sweet taste similar to green peas. High in protein, fiber, isoflavones, and calcium, they are available in Japanese groceries frozen in the pod as *edamamé*. These are boiled or steamed (see page 110) and eaten with salt as a snack—and they are positively addictive! They are now marketed frozen in North America without the pods under the name *sweet beans*, and are also available canned. They can be eaten as a hot vegetable like peas or corn; used in soups, salads, stir-fries, and casseroles; or substituted for lima beans or cooked beans in dips and spreads. You might try growing green soybeans in your garden.

SOYNUTS _____

Soynuts or roasted soybeans are available in natural food stores or the sources on page 184, or you can make your own (page 111). Soaked whole or split dried soybeans are lightly cooked and then roasted in the oven until crunchy like nuts, for which they can be used as a substitute. They have lots of protein, fiber, isoflavones, and calcium, and are lower in fat than nuts, so they make an excellent snack food. They are usually sold salted and can be flavored with various spices and herbs.

SOYNUT BUTTER

Soynut butter is a paste of ground roasted soybeans that is similar to peanut butter but is lower in fat and contains all of the protein, fiber, calcium, and isoflavones of soybeans. It usually contains some salt, sweetener, and oil.

SOYMILK

Soymilk is available in many supermarkets, as well as in natural food stores and Asian markets. It can be used to replace cow's milk in baking and other recipes, as well as on cereal and in hot beverages. To avoid curdling in hot beverages, add your hot coffee or tea to the soymilk, rather than the other way around. Several modern processing techniques make it possible to produce a soymilk with a greater taste appeal than the traditional Asian-style soymilks. Soymilk comes in aseptic cartons with a shelf life of one year or refrigerated in cartons like milk.

Examine the labels of soymilk to see how much protein and fat different brands contain; amounts vary. The higher the protein level, the greater the phytochemical and isoflavone content; look for 4 percent protein if possible. Fat content is 1 to 3 percent. Soymilk is lactose- and cholesterol-free, and now often comes fortified with calcium, vitamin D, and other nutrients. You can buy it plain or flavored with vanilla, almond, carob, or chocolate.

There are also delicious powdered soymilk beverages on the market. These are usually naturally sweetened so that they taste more like cow's milk. Do not confuse them with plain soymilk powder (see below), which is useful for baking, but does not always make a palatable beverage. The better-tasting powdered soymilk beverages can be mixed with less water than is called for on the label to make a soy cream. Or blend them with a little silken tofu to make a cream that is excellent for cooking.

Do not use soymilk in place of infant formula. If you cannot breast-feed, use a specially formulated soy-based infant formula.

SOYMILK POWDER

Soymilk powder is usually found in bulk in natural or natural food stores. It is basically an unflavored dry powder that is useful for baking (and less expensive than liquid soymilk), but it does not always make a palatable beverage. Two tablespoons of soymilk powder combined with one cup water equals one cup of soymilk.

SOY PROTEIN ISOLATE

Soy protein isolate is essentially pure soy protein processed from defatted soy flakes. However, not only the fat but also the soluble and insoluble sugars and the fiber are removed. What remains is 90 percent pure protein, some residual minerals, and a trace of fat. The powder is bland and highly digestible, and is easy to add to shakes and other recipes. It can be used as an emulsifier, to bind fat and water together, and it lends a creamy texture if used in the correct amount. Too much can turn your recipe to cement.

New processing techniques have created a powder that contains high levels of isoflavones, which can vary from 15 to 103 milligrams per ounce. Not only does this depend on the brand you buy, but there will also be some variations within the same brand; manufacturers will often list an average amount on their products. The amount of isoflavones in soybeans can vary somewhat due to crop conditions, variety of bean, etc., and the standards used to measure isoflavones are still being established. Nonetheless, there are still brands which stand out among the crowd; Solgar Iso-Soy Powder, GeniSoy's UltraSoy Protein Powder, and Take Care Soy Protein Powder all have high levels of isoflavones. Soy protein isolate can be purchased in natural food stores, supplement stores, and from the sources on page 184. Plain or flavored versions are available. They keep very well without refrigeration.

TEXTURED SOY PROTEIN

Textured soy protein (TVP® or textured vegetable protein, as it is sometimes called) is processed by mixing defatted soy flour with water, cooking it at high pressure, then extruding the cooked mixture through a machine that makes a variety of textured and shaped products. The extrusion process causes the unique meat-like texture. Sometimes it is flavored before extrusion, but the unflavored varieties are more widely available in natural food stores and from the sources on page 184. It is used primarily in a granular form to replace ground meat or in chunk form in stews and kebabs. There is even a "chiken brest" available now, good breaded and baked, or for dishes such as Italian-style scaloppine. You can also get organic varieties of textured soy. (See sources on page 184.)

Textured soy protein is a low-fat, inexpensive dry product. It is not the same thing as hydrolyzed plant protein or soy isolate, and unflavored varieties contain no MSG or other additives. It has the advantage of being chewier and lower in fat than tofu and can take the place of frozen tofu in many recipes. Even if you object to using meat alternatives on a regular basis, it makes a great transitional food for people who are accustomed to eating meat and, despite the best of motives and intentions, miss those familiar flavors and, especially, textures. I have had great success in serving textured soy protein dishes to nonvegetarians. Textured soy protein chunks have such a meaty texture that, when cooked in a flavorful mixture, I have had anxious vegetarians ask me if I'm sure their food includes no meat!

Unreconstituted textured soy protein will keep for a long time. It has no cholesterol and almost no fat or sodium, and it is an excellent source of protein and fiber. It is easily rehydrated for use in soups, stews, casseroles, and sauces. In fact, if your mixture is very brothy, you can just add the textured soy protein in its dry state, and it will absorb the flavorful broth.

The granules are quickly hydrated by mixing them with an almost equal amount of very hot or boiling liquid, covering, and then letting them stand for five minutes or so. Water is fine if the granules are to be added to a spicy mixture, but you also can use a flavorful broth or tomato juice, or add a tablespoon or two of light soy sauce or a teaspoon of yeast extract (see page 59) to the hot water. The general rule is ⅞ cup liquid to each cup of textured soy protein granules. This yields about 1¾ cups.

The chunks and brests take a little longer to reconstitute, but have an amazingly meat-like texture and a pleasant, mild flavor. Besides stews, the chunks can be used in stir-fries and kebabs, and can be deep-fried. Both the chunks and brests can be oven-fried by coating with Seasoned Flour, page 144, and baking at 400°F for about 10 minutes per side.

Reconstitute the chunks by simmering 1½ cups dry chunks in 3 cups water with 3 tablespoons soy sauce, 3 tablespoons ketchup or tomato paste, and 1 tablespoon nutritional yeast flakes (optional) for 15 to 30 minutes, depending upon how tender you like them. Cool and store in the cooking broth. I usually make four or more times this amount and freeze it in two-cup portions for quick meals later on. Drain the chunks before using them, and pat them dry before coating with flour, frying, or marinating. The brests should be simmered for 30 to 40 minutes until tender, then drained and prepared like the chunks.

When I'm substituting for meat in a recipe, I figure that one pound of meat is equal to about two cups of reconstituted granules or chunks.

SOY MEAT ALTERNATIVES _____

Soy meat alternatives are now available in literally hundreds of brands and forms in natural food stores and supermarkets around the world. They usually contain tofu or tempeh, textured soy protein, and soy concentrates and/or isolates, and they may also contain some seitan (wheat gluten). These new products take the shape of hamburgers, ground beef, hot dogs, sausage, deli meats or cold cuts, pepperoni for pizza, meatballs, ham or Canadian bacon (back bacon), and poultry cutlets or nuggets. Many are very low in fat and can be either frozen or refrigerated. They usually require only heating, not cooking. Some brands may contain egg products, but most are vegan; read the labels. Many brands are delicious and are available in supermarkets, where they are purchased not only by vegetarians but by omnivorous shoppers who want to lower fat and cholesterol in their diets.

TOFU

Tofu (or bean curd, soybean curd, or doufu) in many varieties is available widely these days. It can best be described as a soft cheese-like food made from soymilk that is curdled with mineral salts and then drained and pressed into different textures. It is used widely in Asian cooking and vegetarian cooking. This isoflavone-rich soyfood is extremely versatile, taking on flavors easily, and can be used to substitute for dairy products, meat, poultry, seafood, and eggs.

Most supermarkets and natural food stores carry several different types of tofu. You may find soft tofu, used mainly for drinks and desserts; medium-firm, the Japanese style; firm, the Chinese style; or extra-firm, also called pressed, which is excellent for marinating, stir-frying, and making kebabs. Dessert tofu is a soft tofu that is sweetened and flavored and often served cubed with fruit. It can be used in puddings, shakes, and frozen desserts. You may find some varieties of tofu in bulk in large tubs of water or in vacuum-packed plastic tubs. Tofu that is opened should be covered with fresh water daily and kept in a sealed container in the refrigerator.

You can freeze medium-firm to extra-firm tofu for 48 hours or more. When you thaw it out and squeeze out the water, it takes on a very chewy texture. This makes a great hamburger replacement in chili, spaghetti sauces, sloppy Joes, and casseroles.

In Asian markets and some large supermarkets, you can find Chinese five-spice tofu, which is pressed tofu marinated in a flavorful mixture, good for stir-fries. You will also find some Japanese varieties of fried tofu, such as *aburage*, or flat sheets of fried tofu that can be made into stuffed pouches, rolled around fillings, or cut into strips for soup. You may also find cubes or triangles of golden deep-fried tofu called *atsuage*, which are excellent for stir-fries, barbecue sauces, sweet and sour dishes, curry mixtures, kebabs, and many other uses. Although these are fried, boiling water is poured over them and most of the oil squeezed out. These varieties are very concentrated sources of protein and isoflavones.

In Asian markets you may also be able to find jars of Chinese fermented tofu or *doufu-ru*. This comes in a white variety, a hot, spicy version, and a red version. It is used as a condiment in China to add richness to sauces and marinades. The white variety has a taste similar to that of blue cheese. It keeps for a long time in the refrigerator.

There are many modern varieties of tofu available, including smoked tofu, baked tofu, and marinated tofu. These can replace meats, poultry, and even smoked fish in stir-fries, sautés, casseroles, salads and sandwiches.

In addition, you can find silken tofu, which is sold in aseptic packages and keeps for about a year unopened. It is made right in the package by adding a curdling agent to a richer, thicker soymilk than that used for regular tofu. Silken tofu comes in soft, firm, and extra-firm varieties, as well as regular and low-fat. It is wonderful for blended, creamy mixtures, such as puddings, sauces, soups, and pie fillings.

For an excellent overview of tofu, read *The Book of Tofu: Food for Mankind* by William Shurtleff and Akiko Aoyagi (Ten Speed Press, 1998).

TEMPEH

Tempeh (pronounced tem-pay) is a cultured soybean product, sometimes containing other beans and grains, that originated in Indonesia. It has a slightly nutty taste and firm texture that many people like as a meat or poultry substitute, especially in stir-fry dishes. It can be marinated, baked, grilled, and deep-fried. (Fried tempeh is quite delicious.) It is a good source of soy protein, soy fiber, and isoflavones, and it is easy to digest.

It is usually available frozen in eight-ounce packages—about four servings—or as a marinated cutlet in the refrigerator section of natural foods stores. It should be kept frozen after purchasing and should be fried or steamed before adding to a dish for which no other cooking is required.

Check out *The Book of Tempeh: A Super Soyfood from Indonesia* by William Shurtleff and Akiko Aoyagi (Harper and Row, 1979), and *The Tempeh Cookbook* by Dorothy R. Bates (1989) from the Book Publishing Company.

SOYBEAN SAUCES & PASTES

Hoisin sauce, Chinese black bean sauce, Chinese brown bean sauce, and Szechuan hot bean paste all contain soy. (Chinese fermented black beans, from which black bean sauce is made, are actually black soybeans.)

These popular Chinese condiments are readily available in jars or cans in Asian grocery stores or the Asian section of large supermarkets. They keep indefinitely when refrigerated.

YUBA

Bean-curd skin or yuba is considered a delicacy in China and Japan. It is made by simmering soymilk and lifting off the skin that forms on the top, just like that on dairy milk. This skin can be used fresh, or it can be dried in sheets or rolled-up sticks. The sticks are used in soups, stews, and stir-fries, and can also be barbecued. The sheets can be cut up like noodles, or used in soups, stews, and stir-fries as well. They can be rolled around fillings and baked, steamed, or fried for delicious appetizers, or used as a crispy skin around vegetarian poultry substitutes. Yuba is a very concentrated soyfood. The dried version, available in Asian markets and some large supermarkets, must be soaked in warm water before using.

SOY SAUCE

Soy sauce, shoyu, and tamari are fermented soy products that lend a rich, meaty flavor to vegetarian as well as Asian recipes. Shoyu is the Japanese word for soy sauce; tamari is actually the dark liquid by-product of the miso-making process. It is delicious—and expensive. Most of what is labeled tamari is actually just a naturally brewed soy sauce.

Do not use cheap soy sauce that contains hydrolyzed vegetable protein and caramel coloring. Most supermarkets carry naturally brewed, inexpensive Chinese and Japanese soy sauce in light, dark, and mushroom varieties. *Lite* means that less salt is used. The label should state that it contains only soybeans, salt, water, and sometimes wheat.

MISO

Miso is a Japanese fermented soybean-and-grain paste usually made with rice or barley, which is used as a soup base, similar to bouillon paste or cubes, and flavoring. It is salty but highly nutritious and valued for its digestive properties. Unpasteurized miso contains beneficial bacteria similar to that in yogurt, so it should be added to cooked foods at the last minute and not brought to the boiling point. Natural food stores generally carry a number of varieties: dark, light, yellow, red, sweet, and so on.

I generally use a light brown rice or barley miso, which is made the old-fashioned way right here on Denman Island, British Columbia, by master miso-maker Yoshi Yoshihara (Shinmeido Miso brand), but you can use a sweet white, mellow white, or mellow beige miso in my recipes. In vegetarian foods, miso lends a fermented cheesy flavor.

Read more about this wonderful food in *The Book of Miso* by William Shurtleff and Akiko Aoyagi (Autumn Press, 1976).

SOY CHEESE ALTERNATIVES _____

Soy cheese alternatives are not something I use very often, and they are not a dependable source of isoflavones. I use Soymage 100 percent nondairy Parmesan substitute, which is tofu-based and calcium-enriched. It is quite delicious and will keep in the refrigerator for six months, even longer in the freezer. I substitute about half as much of it for the Parmesan called for in recipes.

Soymage also makes an acceptable vegan mozzarella substitute called Soychunk Italian Flavor, which tastes pretty good—more like a Swiss cheese, actually—and melts pretty well.

OTHER VEGETARIAN FOODS TO BE FAMILIAR WITH

Two other foods that I use often in my recipes are nutritional yeast and yeast extract. Both add rich flavor and many B vitamins to soyfoods. Nutritional yeast is an inactive food yeast grown on a molasses base. It comes in the form of either a golden powder or golden flakes. You can sprinkle it on top of food or add to food when you cook to give a golden

---

Putting the Brakes on Gas

Most people have no trouble with soy products except perhaps for whole soybeans, roasted soybeans (soynuts), and soy flour. Still, there is considerable variability in reactions, and some people are very uncomfortable after eating soyfoods.

Intestinal gas is caused by certain sugars found in soy, namely, raffinose and stachyose. Humans lack an enzyme called alpha-galactosidase, which is necessary to process these sugars. Instead, they enter the lower intestines intact, where they are metabolized by bacteria, which produce gases such as carbon dioxide, hydrogen, and even methane. The variations in the level of discomfort a person experiences may be because people have different levels of bacterial flora in the lower intestine.

Fermented soy products such as tempeh, miso, natto, and soy sauce, are almost devoid of gas-producing qualities because the bacteria that are part of the fermentation process have already digested the sugars.

If you have a lot of gas after eating whole soy products, you may want

---

color and cheesy flavor. It can be found in most natural food stores or from the sources on page 184.

Yeast extract is better known as Marmite or Vegemite and is popular in Canada and the British Isles as a spread for toast. With its distinctively dark and earthy flavor, its use as a stand-alone food is an acquired taste. But as a complementary flavoring for soyfoods, it really comes into its own, providing rich flavor similar to soy sauce, but with more complexity. If you can find this in speciality stores or large markets in your area, it may soon become your favorite ingredient when a beef-like flavor is needed. See page 184 for mail order sources if you cannot find it in your area.

Second-generation soyfoods (soy frozen desserts, puddings, mayonnaise, sour cream, etc.) abound in natural food stores. You can find tofu mayonnaise and salad dressings, tofu sour cream and cream cheese, tofu-based dips and pâtés, soy-based frozen desserts, puddings, frozen dinners and pizzas, soups, and many other specialty foods. Although most of these are excellent foods, they cannot be depended upon for isoflavones, protein, and other nutrients. Their soy content may be lower than less processed soy products.

---

to stick to the concentrated soy protein products, including soy protein isolate; textured soy concentrates (similar to other textured soy, but with a lower carbohydrate content); and tofu or the fermented products mentioned previously. Or try Beano, a liquid enzyme that you sprinkle on food before eating; it works well for many people. Some people swear by adding the sea vegetable kombu while cooking soybeans, or using digestive spices such as ginger, cumin, and fennel.

Finally, keep in mind that flatulence may actually have benefits. Bifidobacteria, a friendly and naturally occurring bacteria in the human gut, is believed by many scientists to play a very important role in the health of the colon. Bifidobacteria use raffinose and stachyose as a source of nutrition; these undigested sugars give bifidobacteria a good chance of surviving over harmful bacteria. Breast-fed babies have high levels of bifidobacteria in their intestines, which may be one reason that they are more resistant to infection than bottle-fed babies. Some Japanese scientists believe that people with high levels of bifidobacteria in their colons live longer. Also, high numbers of bifidobacteria may be linked to reduced carcinogens in human feces.

Chapter 6

Baking and cooking with soyfoods

Are you soyphobic? Do you or any member of your family suffer from fear of tofu? These are not uncommon conditions in the Western world, but they are not insurmountable. When I hear, "Yuck! I hate tofu!" or see that grimace when I talk about the goodness of soyfoods, I ask people how long it has been since they tasted tofu or soymilk, and in what form they tried it. Subjects often reveal they have never tasted any soy—at least, not knowingly—and it is merely the thought of eating that soft, white, jiggly cube that repels. Just as often, I determine that tofu was tried only once, floating limply in a soup in an Oriental restaurant, or that soymilk or a soy meat analog was tried twenty years ago, when these products tasted so terrible that only the most devoted vegetarian would eat them, and then only out of necessity!

I might gently ask whether the person dislikes liver, raw oysters, caviar, or anything else that I find disgusting. Usually, they do eat a few of these things. Then I ask what they have against a food made from a nice clean soybean that does not have any slimy, smelly innards. This often gets them to think of tofu in a different light. Then I explain that tofu is a bland food, sort of like flour, that very few people eat plain. Even the Japanese eat it this way only when it is absolutely fresh; you have to do things with tofu. I tell them that it doesn't have to be soft and jiggly, that they would probably love the pressed or extra-firm variety, marinated in a tasty soy mixture and stir-fried or crisply pan-fried with a coating. I explain that there are new soy products available in supermarkets today that taste so close to dairy milk, burgers, wieners, and ham that even meat-loving teenagers approve of them.

This might pique the subject's interest enough to try a recipe or two, or to buy a packet of soy deli slices, but there is nothing like offering a selection of home-cooked soy dishes to really win over a soyphobic. I like nothing better than to invite some friends over for dinner, have them rave over this dish or that, then tell them that it was made from tofu or it contained soymilk, not dairy milk, or that it was textured soy protein, not meat, in the stew!

If *you* are the soyphobic, please try some of the recipes in this book. I guarantee that you will find something to like. You'll find many easy ideas for painlessly adding soy to your menus, without even using recipes!

My husband's favorite recipe from early on was Breast of Tofu (page 144), which can be used instead of chicken. My son was won over by Tofu Chocolate Mousse (page 166). He used to call tofu "toad food"! The Tofu-Cashew Cheesecake (page 172-73) and my tofu-based Spanikopita (page 130-31) have converted dozens at a time at potlucks!

So read on, and have fun experimenting. You won't necessarily like everything, but you'll find plenty to cure you of soyphobia or fear of tofu for life!

Baking with soy – converting recipes

TO REPLACE EGGS WITH SOY:

If there are one or two eggs or two to four *unbeaten* egg whites in the recipe, simply substitute ¼ cup regular or low-fat soymilk for each egg. You can mix in a tablespoon of soy protein isolate powder for each egg. You might also like to add a tablespoon of nutritional yeast flakes per egg to add a golden color and extra nutrition. This works in yeast breads, muffins and other quick breads, in simple cakes, and some cookies (see note on cookies, page 64). I think this is a more convenient method than using blended tofu, as some cooks recommend, and I believe it produces better results, but you can try it both ways.

If the recipe calls for one or two *beaten* egg whites, substitute two teaspoons powdered egg replacer (available at natural food stores or from the sources on page 184) mixed with two tablespoons water per egg white. Beat with an electric mixer until the mixture is very frothy and holds a soft peak. (It won't hold a stiff peak the way egg white does.) Fold this into batters just as you would beaten egg white.

For yeast breads, you may have to add 1½ tablespoons powdered egg replacer as well as ¼ cup soymilk per egg to bread machine recipes.

For glazing baked goods without eggs, simply brush on soymilk. This makes a lovely golden-brown finish.

Notes on leavening: You don't need more leavening when you eliminate eggs from baking. Use only 1 teaspoon baking powder per cup of flour or, if using sour soymilk or other acid ingredient, ½ teaspoon baking soda per cup of flour. Too much leavening can destroy vitamins and leave an unpleasant aftertaste.

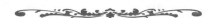

To replace milk and milk products with soy:

Buttermilk: Use either soymilk curdled with lemon juice or vinegar (about 1 tablespoon per cup of soymilk), soy yogurt thinned with some soymilk, or Soy Buttermilk (page 87);

Cheese:

    Soymage Nondairy Soychunk

    Soymage Nondairy Parmesan Substitute,

    Bechamel Sauce (page 96-97)

    some of the variations of Tofu-Cashew Cream Cheese (pages 94-95)

    Melty Soy Pizza Cheese (page 103)

    Quick Tofu Feta and variations (page 106-07)

Cottage cheese: Use Tofu Cottage Cheese (page 93);

Cream: Use a commercial liquid soy coffee creamer, a rich soymilk, or Soy Cream (page 99);

Cream cheese or mascarpone: Use Tofutti's Better Than Cream Cheese or our homemade versions (pages 94 and 99);

Granulated skim milk powder: Use half as much soymilk powder or soy protein isolate powder;

Milk: Use regular or low-fat soymilk, or soymilk powder mixed with water (2 tablespoons powder to 1 cup water);

Ricotta: Use Italian-Style Tofu Ricotta (page 95), or Quick Tofu Ricotta Cheese (page 93);

Sour cream: Use Tofutti's Better Than Sour Cream or our homemade version (page 97);

Yogurt: Use soy yogurt (commercial or homemade, page 86) or Tofu Yogurt (page 97);

Other substitution tips:

To lower the fat: Because the gluten in wheat becomes tough if not coated with fat, low-fat baked goods should be made with at least half pastry flour (white or whole wheat), which has less gluten than all-purpose flour. You may prefer to use all pastry flour. Or experiment with using half wheat flour and half low-gluten or nongluten grain flours, such as oat, barley, and rice.

Substitute smooth, unsweetened applesauce for about two-thirds to three-quarters of the fat called for. You can freeze applesauce—either homemade or commercial—in small containers with amounts that you use often. This also works in yeast breads.

See the note on page 64 for specifics on lowering fat in cookies. Use these formulas for other substitutions:

1½ cups butter or oil = 1 cup applesauce + 6 tablespoons to ½ cup oil or margarine

1 cup butter or oil = ⅔ cup applesauce + ⅓ cup oil or margarine

¾ cup butter or oil = ½ cup applesauce + 4 tablespoons oil or margarine

⅔ cup oil or butter = ½ cup applesauce + 3 tablespoons oil or margarine

½ cup butter or oil = ⅓ cup applesauce + 3 tablespoons oil or margarine

⅓ cup butter or oil = ¼ cup applesauce + 2 tablespoons oil or margarine

¼ cup butter or oil = 3 tablespoons applesauce + 1½ tablespoons oil or margarine

Working with unbleached sugar: Sift Sucanat or dark unbleached sugar, then mix it or any coarse sugar, such as turbinado, with the liquid ingredients, preferably in a blender. If you want to mix coarse sugar with the dry ingredients, it should be blended in a dry blender with a little of the flour from the recipe, until it is more powdery and will mix well with the dry ingredients. Otherwise, it may sink to the bottom of a thin batter.

For a tender crumb: Mix 2 parts pastry flour, 1 part regular flour, and 1 part regular or low-fat soy flour. For instance, if a recipe calls for 2 cups of flour, substitute 1 cup of pastry flour mixed with ½ cup regular flour and ½ cup soy flour. (I like to use whole-wheat pastry flour with unbleached white flour, but you could use regular whole-wheat flour with white cake and pastry flour, if that is easier to obtain.) More soy flour than this can affect the taste and color of the finished product.

A note on recipes with blended tofu

When a recipe calls for blending or processing tofu until very smooth, that is exactly what it means! You must be patient and let the mixture blend until there is no grainy texture left. This may take several minutes, especially if your machine is not very efficient. Keep testing and scraping down the sides occasionally. The reason that I am emphasizing this is that I have had my own recipes prepared by others, and sometimes the whole texture of the dish is ruined by insufficient blending.

Experiment with adding soy protein isolate powder to your baked goods. For instance, add ¼ cup to your recipe for a dozen muffins. You may be able to add more, but proceed cautiously; too much can make a gummy product.

For cookies: Follow the same general advice for baking with soy, except instead of egg replacer, you can use ¼ cup soymilk for each egg or two unbeaten egg whites, or 1 tablespoon whole flaxseed blended with ¼ cup water for several minutes, until it's the consistency of beaten egg white. (Flaxseed also contains plant estrogens, by the way.)

Replacing the fat in cookies is trickier than in cakes and quick breads, so you'll have to do some experimenting. Using corn syrup instead of applesauce in place of two-thirds to three-quarters of the fat called for in a recipe often works well for cookies. Applesauce makes them softer, and corn syrup makes a crispier product.

Cooking with soy–substituting for meat and other foods

Converting recipes based on animal products to soy-based ones requires some experimentation, but you can easily replace *milk products*; see page 62. Ice cream and other dairy-based frozen desserts can be replaced with the many new brands of soy-based frozen desserts. *Mayonnaise* can be replaced with commercial or homemade Tofu Mayonnaise (page 90) or Soy Mayonnaise (page 91).

In some recipes (particularly Asian ones and soups), you can use *soy noodles* instead of semolina or egg noodles.

Replace *hamburger and sausage* with one of the many soy-based commercial vegetarian burgers, hamburger crumbles, sausages, or burger and sausage mixes on the market today. There are some excellent commercial soy-based vegetarian hot dogs, bacon, Canadian or back bacon, deli slices, pepperoni, and ham in both supermarkets and natural food stores. Experiment with replacing *meat and poultry* with textured soy protein granules and chunks (pages 53-54), tofu and frozen tofu (pages 55-56); commercial baked, smoked, or marinated tofu (try White Wave's Thai-style baked tofu); tempeh (page 56); and yuba (page 57).

Remember that meat substitutes do not add liquid to a dish the way meat does, so you will have to add a little extra liquid when converting meat recipes. Use a flavorful vegetarian broth, wine, soy sauce, tamari, liquid aminos, miso, Marmite or other yeast extract, citrus and other juices, tomato products, more onions, garlic, herbs, and spices, Chinese toasted sesame oil, olive oil, flavorful vinegars such as balsamic, or even a touch of sugar or maple syrup to add flavor to meat-free dishes. And don't neglect the salt; meat and dairy products are naturally salty. See page 31 for information on salt in the diet.

Whole soybeans contain all of the goodness of soy, including the soluble and insoluble fiber that may play a major role in decreasing serum cholesterol levels, but they are not used often in either Western or Asian soy cookery. To many people, the use of cooked dried soybeans smacks of dreary 1970s health-food cooking. However, you can effortlessly add the whole soybean to your meals several times a week, just by making a few substitutions:

Here are ideas for other whole soybean products:

Roasted soybeans (soynuts, page 111) can be used instead of nuts or seeds;

Soynut butter (found commercially prepared in natural food stores or the sources on page 184) instead of peanut butter;

Soy sprouts (page 50) instead of mung bean sprouts. (Soy sprouts should steamed or cooked and not be eaten raw.);

Cooked dried soybeans, available canned, instead of, or in addition to, other varieties of cooked dry beans in bean bakes, pâtés, bean patties, fritters and filled pastries, soups, casseroles, etc.;

Green soybeans (or *sweet beans*), now available in the frozen vegetable section of some supermarkets as well as frozen in Asian stores or canned in some natural food stores. Use them instead of cooked dry beans, fresh fava or broad beans, or fresh or frozen baby lima beans in salads, soups, dips (how about green soybean hummus?), succotash, casseroles, pasta dishes, and other recipes.

Black soybeans, available canned in natural food stores, instead of black beans in chili, South American-style bean dishes, refried beans and bean dips, gazpacho, and salads. They are very tasty and creamy inside, and actually a chestnut-brown on the outside when cooked.

When cooking dry soybeans, including black soybeans, remember that 1½ cups dry soybeans yield about 4½ cups cooked.

Canned soybeans are a convenience, but cooking your own is certainly cheaper. I usually cook a big batch and freeze it in 2-cup containers. The cooking broth is quite tasty, by the way, and can be used in soups and gravies. Frozen soybeans can be thawed quickly in a microwave oven or in a colander under hot running tap water.

If you can soybeans yourself, pressure can *only* because of their low acid content! Drain the soaked beans and bring them to a boil with fresh water or vegetarian broth. Boil two minutes, skimming off the foam. Fill sterilized pint canning jars with hot soaked soybeans to within an inch of the top, then pour in the hot cooking liquid just to cover. (Larger jars might not reach the proper temperature in the middle.) Drizzle the top of each jar with 1 teaspoon of oil to control foaming. Wipe the tops of the jars with a sterile cloth, then twist on new lids. Pressure can according to directions for your canner for 65 minutes at 10 pounds pressure. Remove the jars from the canner and tighten the seals. Cool thoroughly and remove the rings.

Dry soybeans need to be soaked 6 to 8 hours or overnight in plenty of water. They achieve maximum tenderness when pressure cooked. If you have no pressure cooker, consider freezing the soaked beans in fresh water for at least 48 hours before cooking them; this seems to tenderize them considerably. Drain the soaked soybeans, and cover with fresh water about an inch above the beans. Bring to a boil and boil for about 3 minutes, skimming off the foam, then reduce the heat, cover, and simmer for 3 to 4 hours, or until tender. Add more water if necessary.

You can flavor the water with bay leaf, onion, garlic, celery, salt, and other seasonings you like. Japanese cooks add a strip of dried kombu, a sea vegetable, to soybeans when cooking them, which is supposed to make them more digestible.

To pressure cook, drain and rinse the soaked beans, and place them in a pressure cooker with ample water to cover, taking care not to fill the pot more than two-thirds full. Bring the beans to a boil and simmer for a few minutes, skimming off as much foam and any loose skins as possible. Add any seasonings you may be using and 1 tablespoon of oil for every 1½ cups of dry beans. (The oil controls foaming.) Lock the lid in place and bring up to pressure according to the directions for your pot. Reduce the heat just enough to maintain high pressure, and cook for 45 minutes. Bring the pressure down by placing the pot in the sink and running cold water over the lid.

STEAM-FRYING

One term that you will see over and over in my recipes is steam-fry. It simply means sautéeing or stir-frying with little or no fat. To do this, use a heavy skillet, preferably nonstick, or brush on ½ teaspoon of oil with your fingertips. You also can use a well-seasoned wok, oiled the same way.

Heat the pan over high heat, add your chopped onions or other vegetables, and one or two tablespoons of liquid (water, broth, or wine), depending on the amount of vegetables. Cook over high heat until the liquid starts to evaporate, stirring constantly with a spatula or wooden spoon. Keep doing this until the vegetables are done to your liking, adding just enough liquid to keep the vegetables from sticking to the bottom of the pan—you don't want to stew them!

You can brown onions perfectly with this method. As soon as the natural sugar in the onions starts to brown on the bottom and edges of the pan, add a little liquid and scrape the carmelized residue from the pan, mixing it into the liquids and cooking onions. Keep doing this until the onions are soft and brown, being careful not to scorch them.

Chapter 7

Breakfast foods and beverages

Breakfast is an excellent meal for introducing soyfoods into your diet, and it is perhaps the meal most in need of revamping in North America. Millions of North Americans eat no breakfast at all, making them vulnerable later in the morning to the temptations of doughnut shops, sugary coffee, cola drinks, and candy bars in a vain attempt to fend off the fatigue and crankiness that signals low blood sugar. Many others start the day with fatty repasts of fried eggs, bacon, ham, or sausage—often accompanied by fried potatoes, buttered toast, or pancakes dripping butter and artificial syrup—which cause sluggishness and clog the arteries.

A light breakfast containing fruit, whole grains, and some type of soy protein is easily digested and contains enough protein, fiber, and complex carbohydrates to keep you alert, energetic, and productive until your lunch break. This type of breakfast can be as simple as a soy-fruit shake or fresh fruit and soy yogurt with whole-grain toast, or a bowl of commercial whole-grain cereal and soymilk with fruit. You may require a more substantial meal, but it does not have to be loaded with refined carbohydrates and saturated fats in order to be hearty.

The easiest way to begin redesigning breakfast is to experiment with all of the delicious new soymilks available in supermarkets and natural food stores and find the one you like best. Many are now fortified with calcium, vitamin D, and other nutrients. Some people like it rich and creamy; others prefer a "lite" version, especially if they are used to low-fat or fat-free dairy milk. I prefer to buy plain soymilk and flavor it myself, but vanilla, almond, carob, and chocolate soymilks are all available commercially in quart or liter cartons, individual-size aseptic cartons, and two-quart cartons. You can even buy a product called Yogi Tea, a spicy, milky Indian tea (see page 89 for a homemade version), and milky coffee beverages (see page 85) made with soymilk in cartons.

You may even find a powdered version that you prefer. It's a good idea to keep some powdered soymilk around the house, in any case, to use as you would skim milk powder in baking and fortifying other foods. The powder doesn't make a beverage that tastes as good as fresh soymilk, but it's fine for baking and many other recipes. For drinking, you will need a good-tasting type that probably contains some sweetener.

Once you have found a brand of soymilk that you like, start using it instead of dairy milk. If you don't take to soymilk right away, try mixing it half-and-half with dairy milk at first, and gradually increase the amount of soymilk in the mix. Or do as my husband did and just make a commitment to try it for a month. After a month he thought cow's milk tasted like "the cow had put her foot in the bucket"! He now prefers soymilk even in his cappuccinos.

Ways to use soymilk for breakfast:

1) Use it to make beverages. Make cocoa and other hot milky drinks with it (pages 83-85 and 89). Make fruit smoothies and shakes with it (page 80). Use it in coffee, tea, latte, and frothy cappuccino (page 85). If you are used to cream in coffee, try using a commercial liquid soy coffee creamer, or the richest soymilk you can find instead of cream, gradually replacing it with a lower-fat brand. Blending a tablespoon of soy protein isolate powder to a cup of low-fat soymilk will also make it creamier.
2) Use soymilk on hot and cold cereals.
3) Use soymilk as the liquid in crêpe, pancake, waffle, quick bread, and coffee cake recipes. I also use ¼ cup soymilk in place of each egg called for in quick bread and coffee cake recipes.
4) Use it in yeast breads. They rise to new heights with the special dough-conditioning qualities of soymilk. Substitute ¼ cup soymilk per egg in yeast bread recipes. For bread machine recipes you may have to add 1¼ tablespoon powdered egg replacer per egg as well.
5) Soak bread for French toast in rich vanilla-flavored soymilk instead of the egg-and-milk mixture. A half cup of soymilk is enough for two large, firm slices of bread. I add a dash of vanilla and some freshly grated nutmeg to the soymilk, but you can use a commercial vanilla- or almond-flavored soy drink too.
6) Make your own soy yogurt, soy buttermilk, and soy yogurt cheese with soymilk (pages 86-87).

Basic Tofu Omelet Batter

Yield: 4 large or 8 small omelets

Here is the basic vegan omelet batter and some of my favorite ways to use it. Feel free to substitute your own favorite vegetables and herbs. You can also top with a sauce, such as Italian or Mexican-style tomato sauce, a tofu sour cream-based sauce, or your favorite vegetable-based sauce. This eggless version has excellent flavor, texture, and even an egg-like color. The batter looks very pale, but becomes a darker yellow when cooked.

Per large omelet: Calories 130, Protein 12 g, Soy Protein 8 g, Fat 5 g, Carbohydrates 9 g

1 pound medium-firm tofu

6 tablespoons unbleached white flour or ¼ cup brown rice flour

¼ cup nutritional yeast flakes

1 tablespoon water, dry white wine, marsala, or dry sherry

1 teaspoon baking powder

½ teaspoon salt

½ teaspoon turmeric

¼ teaspoon white pepper

Tofu Omelets, Foo Yung, and Frittate (Italian Baked Omelets)

Tofu makes an excellent stand-in for eggs, and this simple, versatile omelet batter is a prime example. It can be used for individual folded French- or American-style omelets with or without a filling; thicker Italian frittate; and delectable oven-fried tofu foo yung, the little Chinese vegetable omelets usually fried in oil. For French- or American-style omelets, cook one side a little less, so that it doesn't get quite as crispy and make the omelet harder to fold.

Preheat the oven to 500°F.

Blend all the ingredients in a food processor until very smooth. Oil 2 cookie sheets. For each omelet, pour ¼ cup to ½ cup of the batter on the cookie sheet, and spread the batter to make the rounds as thin as possible without making holes. Don't make them too thick; they puff up during cooking. Bake for 6 minutes or until browned and slightly crispy on the bottom. Flip the omelets over and cook another 4 minutes, or until golden brown on the other side. Remove and serve plain or filled with your favorite filling or one of the variations that follow.

❧ Top with chopped vegetarian ham or Canadian or back bacon, sautéed mushrooms or other vegetables, and Melty Soy Pizza Cheese (page 103), soy Parmesan, or grated soy cheese. Fold the omelet around the filling, and serve.

❧ *Denver Omelet:* Add 4 green onions, chopped, 1 green pepper, seeded and chopped, and ½ cup chopped vegetarian ham or Canadian or back bacon to the batter before cooking.

❧ *Tofu Foo Yung:* Add 4 ounces raw mung bean sprouts, chopped, or finely shredded cabbage or carrots, 4 green onions, chopped, and 8 medium mushrooms, chopped, to the batter before cooking. Top with Chinese Brown Sauce.

Chinese Brown Sauce: Combine 1½ cups vegetable broth, 2 tablespoons soy sauce, 1 tablespoon dry sherry or 2 teaspoons vinegar (optional), 2 teaspoons sugar or molasses, and 1½ tablespoon scornstarch dissolved in 1½ tablespoons cold water in a small saucepan. Stir over high heat until thickened and clear.

To microwave, mix the ingredients in a 1-quart microwaveable container. Cook 1 to 2 minutes; whisk and cook 2 minutes more.

Other ways to use soyfoods at breakfast:

1) Soymilk powder, soy flour, tofu, and soy protein isolate powder can also be added to many of the breakfast recipes (see Chapter 6, Baking and Cooking with Soyfoods).
2) If you prefer to buy yogurt, there are several good brands of soy yogurt on the market; try them all, then decide which you prefer. Soy yogurt with fruit and toast makes an excellent, fast, and easy breakfast. Or mix the soy yogurt with fruit to make a breakfast smoothie (page 80).
3) You'll find a few excellent, low-fat soy-based breakfast sausages and bacon slices in food stores. Substitute them for the fatty animal products. They are delicious!
4) In the next chapter, you'll find recipes for soy cheeses and spreads to embellish your breakfast toast, as well as rich-tasting soy creams to pour over fresh fruit.
5) You can cut out cholesterol and add soy to your diet if you replace breakfast eggs with versatile tofu. You can buy a commercial dry scrambler mix in natural food stores that makes an excellent faux tofu scrambled eggs, but it's easy enough to make your own (page 75), as well as tofu-based omelets (pages 70-71), which make elegant brunch fare.

Tofu Crêpes

Yield: 12 to 13 crêpes

These are really excellent. They have that flexible eggy texture of regular crêpes. You can freeze them too.

Per crêpe: Calories 63, Protein 3 g, Soy Protein 2 gm., Fat 1 g, Carbohydrates 9 g

1½ cups soymilk

1 cup unbleached flour or whole-wheat pastry flour

½ cup medium-firm tofu

¼ cup soy flour

1 to 2 tablespoons nutritional yeast flakes (optional)

1 tablespoon sugar

½ teaspoon salt

½ teaspoon baking powder

¼ teaspoon turmeric

A few gratings of nutmeg

Vegetable oil

Process all the ingredients except the vegetable oil in a food processor or blender until very smooth. Heat a nonstick 8-inch skillet over medium-high heat. Pour a small amount of vegetable oil on a paper towel, and wipe the pan lightly. Pour about 3 tablespoons of batter into the pan. Roll and tilt the pan until the batter evenly covers the bottom. Cook for a few seconds until the top looks dry. Carefully loosen the crêpe with a spatula, and flip it over. Cook a few seconds, until the other side is flecked with brown spots. Slide the crêpe onto a plate. Fold into quarters, roll like a jelly roll, or leave flat if you are going to stack crêpes with filling. If you are going to use the crêpes shortly, cover them with a clean tea towel.

Wipe the pan with oil and stir the batter before cooking each crêpe.

Bright Idea: You can make a form of oven pancake called a Dutch baby (don't ask me where the name came from!) with a variation of the crêpe batter. Replace the soymilk, flour, tofu, soy flour, and yeast flakes with:

> 1 cup water
> 1¼ cups unbleached flour
> 1½ cups medium-firm tofu
> 2 tablespoons powdered egg replacer

Use the remaining ingredients as listed. Heat 24 muffin tins in a 450°F oven. Grease each cup with about ¼ teaspoon margarine or oil. Divide the batter evenly among the 24 hot muffin cups. Bake at 450°F for 15 minutes. Reduce the oven temperature to 400°F for 5 minutes. The muffins should puff up in the middle and be brown and somewhat crispy on the outside. Serve with fresh lemon wedges to squirt on them, and top with powdered unbleached sugar (grind in a dry blender with a little cornstarch), maple syrup, or fruit preserves. These even make an acceptable stand-in for Yorkshire pudding! Just leave out the sugar and nutmeg.

72 *Soyfoods Cooking For A Positive Menopause*

Either fill the crêpes and serve, or let them cool and place in a plastic bag or storage container with pieces of waxed paper in between each crêpe. Refrigerate for up to 3 days, or freeze them for future use. (Thaw thoroughly before filling.)

♪ *Dessert Crêpes:* Add 2 tablespoons sugar, 1 teaspoon vanilla, and ½ teaspoon pure orange or lemon extract to the batter. Fill the crêpes with Tofu-Cashew Cream Cheese or one of its variations (pages 94-95) or Tofu Mascarpone (page 99), and top with sweetened fresh fruit, liqueur, and or any sweet sauce.

♪ *Saffron Crêpes:* Add ¼ teaspoon Spanish saffron to the batter.

♪ *Buckwheat Crêpes:* Substitute ½ cup buckwheat flour for ½ cup of the wheat flour and use soured soymilk (add about 1 tablespoon lemon juice to the soymilk) or ¾ cup soy yogurt mixed with ¾ cup soymilk instead of all soymilk.

Fried Egg Tofu

This is a super-easy, delicious egg substitute. Take as many quarter- to half-inch-thick slices of medium-firm tofu as you like. Dredge in nutritional yeast flakes until both sides are coated. Brown the slices over medium-high heat in a nonstick skillet until golden-brown on both sides. Eat plain, or as a sandwich, with ketchup. For a stronger flavor, dip the tofu in soy sauce before dredging in the yeast flakes. This is great for cold sandwiches.

Tofu Frittate

Yield: two 10-inch frittate (12 servings)

Frittate are Italian omelets, which are thick and firm—more akin to the Spanish "tortilla" or Persian kuku than to soft French folded omelets. They are usually full of vegetables and often contain potatoes or leftover pasta as well. The traditional way to cook a frittata is in a skillet on top of the stove, but this simple tofu mixture works better in the oven.

Frittate are usually served at room temperature, and they make an excellent between-meal snack, eaten either out of hand or on a piece of crusty bread—great for picnic food! Frittate are wonderful make-ahead brunch fare too.

Per serving: Calories 154, Protein 10 g, Soy Protein 6 g., Fat 3 g, Carbohydrates 20 g

2 tablespoons extra-virgin olive oil

One batch Basic Tofu Omelet Batter (pages 70-71)

1 large onion, thinly sliced

2 medium cooked potatoes, peeled and sliced, or 1 cup leftover cooked pasta (with or without sauce)

Freshly ground black pepper

About 2 tablespoons soy Parmesan

Add the following to the batter at the same time you add the cooked onions. Use any combination you wish to make a total of 1 to 2 cups.

1 tablespoon to ⅓ cup chopped fresh herbs, such as Italian parsley, basil, mint, or sage

Chopped vegetarian bacon, ham, Canadian bacon, sausage, or pepperoni

Sliced black Italian olives

Chopped sun-dried tomatoes

Thinly sliced artichoke hearts

2 cloves garlic, minced

½ cup chopped, cooked bitter greens, such as arugula, dandelion, endive, or borage

Thinly sliced bell pepper

Thinly sliced zucchini or summer squash

Other vegetables, cooked until tender-crisp and cut in small pieces: asparagus, broccoli, cauliflower, mushrooms, green beans, or eggplant

Preheat the oven to 450°F.

Pour 1 tablespoon olive oil in each of two 10-inch cast-iron skillets or baking dishes, and place them in the oven while it heats up. When the oil is hot, add the onion to the pans. Bake for about 5 minutes. Add the onion to the Basic Tofu Omelet Batter. Add the potatoes or pasta to the batter, and mix well.

Lower the oven temperature to 350°F. Dividing the batter evenly, pour it into the two skillets and spread evenly to the edges. Sprinkle with black pepper and soy Parmesan, and bake for 30 minutes.

Remove the pans and cool on racks for 10 minutes. Then loosen the bottom of the frittate, and cut each into 6 pieces. Serve warm or at room temperature. Store leftovers covered in the refrigerator.

My Quick and Easy Scrambled Tofu

Yield: 1 serving

Scrambled tofu is a quick, easy, inexpensive, and delicious way to replace eggs and add soy to your morning meal. It also makes a good supper dish, especially with vegetables added.

Per serving: Calories 123, Protein 13 g, Soy Protein 9 gm., Fat 4 g, Carbohydrates 6 g

½ cup medium-firm or firm tofu (depending on how soft you like your scrambles)

1 tablespoon nutritional yeast flakes

1 to 2 teaspoons soy sauce, or to taste

⅛ teaspoon turmeric

⅛ teaspoon onion powder

Pinch of garlic granules

Salt and pepper, to taste

Chopped fresh herbs, such as chives, basil, or rosemary (optional)

Soy bacon bits (optional)

Lightly oil a nonstick skillet, and heat over high heat. Drain the tofu and crumble into the skillet. Add the remaining ingredients and toss with a spatula to mix well. Cook for several minutes, stirring frequently, until the mixture turns a nice scrambled-egg yellow and is as creamy or as dry as you like it. Add soy sauce, salt, and pepper to taste. Sprinkle with fresh herbs and soy bacon bits, if desired.

If you like, you can add sautéed mushrooms, onions, and bell pepper to the cooked mixture.

Fireweed's Deluxe Scrambled Tofu

Yield: 2 to 3 servings

My friend Fireweed is a fellow Denman Islander and a wonderful cook. This scrambled tofu is gobbled up by vegetarians and omnivores with equal enthusiasm.

She writes, "This dish makes a great breakfast dish for company, since it can easily be made in large quantities the day before. In that case, though, I prefer to add the zucchini or peas closer to serving time. For a crowd you can stretch a small jar of medium-hot salsa with a can of crushed tomatoes or a few fresh tomatoes from the garden, chopped fine or left chunky."

Per serving: Calories 315, Protein 21 g, Soy Protein 11 g, Fat 19 g, Carbohydrates 14 g

2 to 3 teaspoons extra-virgin olive oil

½ cup sliced mushrooms (button, shiitake, oyster, or a mixture)

¾ pound firm tofu, well-drained

5 tablespoons lite soy sauce or Bragg's Liquid Aminos

1 large clove garlic, minced or pressed

1 teaspoon EACH fresh chopped basil, thyme, oregano (or ½ teaspoon each dried), or to taste

1 teaspoon onion salt

1 teaspoon turmeric

6 tablespoons nutritional yeast

2 tablespoons frozen peas (preferably organic baby peas or petit pois)

> *Bright Idea:* You can use ¼ cup diced zucchini instead of the peas, if you wish, and/or ¼ cup diced, peeled fresh tomato.

Oil a large, heavy skillet with a tiny bit of olive oil, and heat over medium heat. Add the mushrooms and cover to cook them in their own juices, lifting the lid only to stir occasionally and keep them from sticking. When they are tender and starting to brown, remove the mushrooms to a bowl and set aside.

Add the 2 teaspoons of oil to the pan. Crumble the tofu into the skillet by squeezing it through your fingers. Cook uncovered over medium heat until most of the moisture has evaporated. Keep scraping the pan with a metal spatula to keep from sticking. When the texture is significantly drier, add the soy sauce, garlic, herbs, and seasonings, and mix well.

Sprinkle on the yeast and mix again. Add the mushrooms, along with their juices, and the peas (or other vegetables). Cover and heat thoroughly, then serve immediately with salsa and toast or potatoes.

Simple Soy Shake

Yield: 1 serving

When you're in a hurry and the cupboards are almost bare!

Per serving: Calories 88, Protein 9 g, Soy Protein 8 g, Fat 0 g, Carbohydrates 13 g

½ cup orange juice, preferably
   freshly squeezed

3 ice cubes

1 heaping tablespoon soy protein
   isolate powder

Process all the ingredients in a blender until smooth and frothy.

Soy Buttermilk Drink

Yield: 1 serving

This was another "desperation" invention. I had low blood sugar and had to rush to a dance class, so I mixed this up on impulse and gulped it down. It was good, tasted a little like buttermilk, and kept me going through the dance class!

Per serving: Calories 96, Protein 4 g, Soy Protein 3 g, Fat 2 g, Carbohydrates 15 g

½ cup orange juice or apple juice

½ cup soymilk

Just stir together in a glass, and drink up!

Pineapple-Orange Soy Shake

Yield: 4 servings

Per serving: Calories 142, Protein 6 g, Soy Protein 5 g, Fat 0 g, Carbohydrates 28 g

One 14-ounce can unsweetened crushed pineapple and juice

1½ cups orange juice

1 frozen banana, sliced

¼ cup soy protein isolate powder

½ teaspoon coconut extract

6 ice cubes

Process all the ingredients in a blender until very smooth.

Orange Julia

Yield: 2 servings

This makes a great breakfast, snack, or dessert.

Per serving: Calories 51, Protein 4 g, Soy Protein 3 g, Fat 1 g, Carbohydrates 6 g

¾ cup water

6 tablespoons frozen orange juice

⅓ cup firm or extra-firm silken tofu, or ¼ cup firm or medium-firm tofu

½ teaspoon vanilla extract

5 ice cubes

Pineapple Julia: Substitute pineapple juice concentrate for the orange juice concentrate

Process all the ingredients, except the ice cubes, in a blender until smooth. Add the ice cubes and blend again. Pour into glasses and serve.

Vegan Eggnog

Yield: 10 servings

This nog will please even those who say they don't like soymilk. Not too thick or cloying, it's a very refreshing drink any time of the year. Make the eggnog mix ahead of time, then blend with the ice cubes just before serving.

Per serving: Calories 155, Protein 5 g, Soy Protein 5 g, Fat 2 g, Carbohydrates 15 g

Two 12.3-ounce boxes extra-firm silken tofu

2 cups soymilk or other plain nondairy milk

⅔ cup unbleached sugar, or 1 cup grade A light maple syrup

¼ teaspoon salt

1 cup cold water

1 cup rum, brandy, or apple juice with either flavoring, to taste

4½ teaspoons vanilla

20 ice cubes

Freshly grated nutmeg

Place the tofu and soymilk in a blender with the sugar and salt. Blend until very smooth. Scrape the mixture into a large bowl or pitcher, and whisk in the water, rum or brandy, and vanilla. Mix well, cover, and refrigerate until serving time.

To serve, process half of the mixture in the blender with 10 of the ice cubes until frothy. Repeat with the remaining cubes. Serve in glasses with nutmeg sprinkled on top.

Tofu Shakes

Yield: 2 servings

This nutritious snack is satisfying any time of the day! The mixture also can be frozen in popsicle molds.

Per serving: Calories 178, Protein 6 g, Soy Protein 5 g, Fat 2 g, Carbohydrates 33 g

1 frozen peeled banana, in chunks

1 cup orange or other fruit juice

½ cup firm or extra-firm silken tofu or medium-firm tofu

Large handful of berries or chunks of mango, peach, or other fresh or frozen fruit (optional)

½ teaspoon nondairy acidophilus powder (optional)

½ teaspoon coconut, vanilla, or almond extract (optional)

Sweetener, to taste

Combine all the ingredients in a blender, and process until smooth. Pour into glasses and drink immediately.

Blender Fruit Smoothie

Yield: 1 serving

You can make a thick, creamy soy smoothie without dairy or even tofu.

Per serving: Calories 188, Protein 9 g, Soy Protein 8 g, Fat 0 g, Carbohydrates 36 g

¾ cup orange or other fruit juice of your choice

1 heaping tablespoon soy protein isolate powder

½ frozen banana (peeled before freezing), cut into chunks

Small handful of berries or chunks of mango, peach, or any other fresh or frozen fruit

Sweetener, to taste

¼ teaspoon nondairy acidophilus powder (optional)

¼ teaspoon coconut, almond, or vanilla extract (optional)

Bright Idea: Use commercial soy yogurt instead of fruit juice. Sweeten to taste.

For a piña colada smoothie, use pineapple juice, frozen banana, and pineapple chunks, and add ¼ teaspoon coconut extract. Add a few drops of rum extract if desired.

Combine all the ingredients in a blender, and process until very smooth. Pour into a glass and serve immediately.

Strawberrry-Almond Soy Smoothie

Yield: 2 servings

Per serving: Calories 136, Protein 7 g, Soy Protein 6 g, Fat 5 g, Carbohydrates 6 g

10 medium or 5 large frozen strawberries, chopped

1 cup soymilk

½ cup regular or silken tofu

2 tablespoons unbleached sugar or grade A light maple syrup

¼ to ½ teaspoon pure almond extract

Process all the ingredients in a blender until very smooth.

Lassi

This Indian yogurt and fruit shake makes a refreshing breakfast, snack, or dessert beverage with tropical overtones.

Per serving: Calories 92, Protein 3 g, Soy Protein 3 g, Fat 1 g, Carbohydrates 17 g

½ cup apricot nectar or frozen papaya or pineapple juice concentrate

1 cup cold water

⅓ cup frozen apple juice concentrate or grade A light maple syrup

½ cup silken tofu, medium-firm tofu, or soy yogurt

2 tablespoons lemon or lime juice

¼ teaspoon coconut extract or ground cardamom, nutmeg, or ginger

1 teaspoon nondairy acidophilus powder (optional)

6 ice cubes

Bright Idea: Substitute ⅔ cup ripe, peeled, chopped mango, papaya, or pineapple or canned unsweetened pineapple for the apricot nectar

Place all the ingredients, except the ice cubes, in a blender, and process until smooth. Add the ice cubes and blend again until the ice is finely ground. Pour into glasses and serve immediately.

Triple Soy Chocolate Milkshake

Yield: 2 servings

Go ahead and indulge! Creamy and frosty, but low in fat and rich in soy. For the richest flavor, use Dutch cocoa. Note: If your blender can't process ice cubes, place them in a plastic or burlap bag and crush them with a hammer first.

Per serving: Calories 241, Protein 19 g, Soy Protein 17 g, Fat 5 g, Carbohydrates 29 g

1 cup soymilk
½ cup medium-firm tofu or firm silken tofu
¼ cup soy protein isolate powder
¼ cup unbleached sugar, or to taste
2 tablespoons unsweetened Dutch cocoa powder
1 teaspoon vanilla or ½ teaspoon peppermint extract
10 ice cubes

Combine all the ingredients, except the ice cubes, in a blender, and process until smooth. Add the ice cubes two at a time, blending briefly after each addition. When all are added, blend until the mixture is smooth and thick. Pour into glasses and serve immediately.

Double Soy Banana Shake: If you have no tofu, substitute 1 ripe banana, peeled and cut into chunks.

Strawberry Shake: Omit the cocoa and use a light unbleached sugar (see page 158) or ¼ cup grade A light maple syrup, and add ½ cup sliced fresh or frozen strawberries. Use only ½ teaspoon vanilla.

Vanilla Shake: Omit the cocoa and use light unbleached sugar (see page 158) or ¼ cup grade A light maple syrup. Increase the vanilla to 2 teaspoons.

Easy Nondairy Hot Cocoa

Yield: 1 serving

Of course, you can just heat up your favorite chocolate-flavored soymilk, but we usually have only plain soymilk in the house and flavor it ourselves in different ways. For a dark, rich-tasting brew, use Dutch cocoa; for a milder drink, use regular cocoa powder. Soy protein isolate powder makes this very creamy.

Per serving: Calories 156, Protein 11 g, Soy Protein 11 g, Fat 5 g, Carbohydrates 17 g

1 cup very hot soymilk

½ tablespoon unsweetened cocoa powder

1 tablespoon unbleached sugar

1 tablespoon soy protein isolate powder

¼ teaspoon vanilla, or ⅛ teaspoon almond or peppermint extract

Combine all the ingredients in a blender. Remove the plastic center part of the blender lid, and cover it with a folded tea towel before blending; this prevents steam build-up inside the blender which can cause hot liquid to explode. Blend until smooth. Pour into a mug and serve immediately.

Microwave Option

Use cold soymilk. Pour all the ingredients into a large microwave-safe mug (large enough to prevent boil-overs), and microwave on high for 1½ to 2 minutes. Whisk before serving.

❧ *Mexican Cocoa:* Add a pinch of cinnamon.

❧ *Christmas Breakfast Cocoa:* Use a candy cane as a stir stick.

❧ *Mocha Cocoa:* Add 1 teaspoon instant coffee or coffee substitute.

❧ *Norwegian Cocoa:* Add 1 teaspoon of rum or a few drops of rum extract and a drop of butter-flavor extract.

❧ *Special Cocoa:* Add a tablespoon or so of chocolate, coffee, orange, almond, or other favorite liqueur, brandy, or rum to the cocoa.

Hot Cocoa Mix

Yield: enough mix for 8 cups cocoa

Per cup: Calories 141, Protein 10 g, Soy Protein 9 g, Fat 2 g, Carbohydrates 24 g

1 cup tofu or soy beverage mix (see page 52) or other nondairy milk powder

½ cup soy protein isolate powder

¼ to ⅓ cup unsweetened Dutch cocoa, or to taste

½ cup unbleached sugar, finely ground in a blender or food processor

½ teaspoon salt

In a medium bowl, mix all the ingredients well with a whisk. Store in a covered airtight container.

For each cup of cocoa, mix a scant ⅓ cup of the mix with 1 cup boiling water and ¼ teaspoon vanilla extract or ⅛ teaspoon almond or peppermint extract in a blender. Remove the plastic center part of the blender lid, and cover it with a folded tea towel before blending; this prevents steam build-up inside the blender which can cause hot liquid to explode. Blend until smooth. Use the variations for Easy Nondairy Hot Cocoa (page 83).

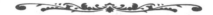

Flavored Hot Soymilk

Heat your favorite soymilk in a small saucepan or the microwave, and sweeten to taste with unbleached sugar or grade A light maple syrup, and add about ¼ teaspoon of pure almond extract or vanilla. Drink as is, or froth it with a plunger-type milk frother or in a blender. (It froths up to about triple in volume, so watch out!)

In India, flavored, frothy hot milks are served for breakfast or as an evening snack. They may be as simple as sweetened milk or milk embellished with spices and nuts. Make a hot soymilk drink as directed above, using almond or coconut extract, but heat the milk with a pinch of cardamom seed or other favorite spice. (Strain out before frothing.) Or sprinkle the top with a little freshly grated nutmeg or ground cinnamon. A tablespoon of sesame tahini can be blended into each cup if you wish. If you like a little jolt of ginger in the morning, blend in 1 to 2 teaspoons grated fresh ginger as well.

Soy Cappuccinos, Lattés, and Iced Coffee Drinks

My husband has a soy cappuccino every morning and now prefers it to the dairy kind. Make it the same way as you would an ordinary cappuccino (espresso with frothed milk), latté (espresso with hot milk), or iced latté over crushed ice), but use regular or low-fat soymilk instead of dairy milk. You may have to try different brands of soymilk to see which one you prefer. We find that soymilk froths up just fine. My husband prefers his coffee made in one of those tiny little Italian stainless-steel stove-top espresso makers, and he now uses one of those great new and inexpensive plunger-type milk frothers, so it isn't necessary to have an expensive machine to make cappuccinos at home. Hot milk also can be frothed, although not quite as well, in a blender.

I recommend organic, naturally decaffeinated coffee, and be sure to use a dark roast that's freshly ground, such as French or Italian.

➤ *Vietnamese Coffee:* For this icy and refreshing drink, make a strong espresso (resulting in about 6 tablespoons of espresso per person), and mix it with 2 tablespoons Sweetened Condensed Soymilk (page 161) per serving. Pour over a tall glassful of rough-crushed ice, about 6 cubes per glass. Serve with a straw. Delicious!

➤ *Cappuccino Milkshakes:* Pour one serving of cooled espresso into a blender, and blend with about ½ cup cold plain, vanilla, carob, or chocolate soymilk and a big scoop of soy frozen dessert in any flavor that goes well with coffee (see pages 176-77). When smooth, pour into a tall glass, and serve with a straw.

➤ *Cappuccino Shake:* For an easier, lower-fat version, blend one serving of cooled espresso (sweeten to taste, if you like) with ⅓ to ½ cup cold soymilk (plain, vanilla, carob, or chocolate), 1 tablespoon soy protein isolate powder, and 3 or 4 ice cubes until frothy and thick. You can also freeze the espresso in ice cubes and blend them with soymilk and sweetener to taste.

➤ *Mocha Latté:* Make a latté using your favorite chocolate-flavored soymilk.

Thick Homemade *Soy Yogurt*

Yield: 1 quart

There are several very good brands of soy yogurt available for yogurt lovers, but if you'd like to try your hand at making inexpensive, creamy, and thick home-made soy yogurt, try this recipe.

Soy protein isolate powder makes all the difference in the creaminess and thickness of the yogurt, as well as adding extra isoflavones, so don't leave it out! Make sure that all your cooking utensils and equipment are sterilized with boiling water, and try to use metal, glass, or rigid plastic.

Use two sterilized pint canning jars to incubate the yogurt. I find the most convenient place to keep the yogurt warm is in one of those inexpensive foam ice chests or portable coolers with a one-quart jar of very hot water placed inside.

Per cup: Calories 128, Protein 16 g, Soy Protein 16 g, Fat 5 g, Carbohydrates 5 g

½ cup soy protein isolate powder

4 cups soymilk*

2 tablespoons unpasteurized, plain, agar-free commercial soy yogurt

*Ideally, use soymilk straight from an unopened package. If you use soymilk that is homemade or from a partially used, refrigerated carton, you must first scald the soymilk, then cool it to room temperature.

Scald any equipment that will come into contact with the mixture, such as the blender jar, spoons, and storage container. Mix the soy protein powder with 2 cups of the soymilk until smooth but not too frothy, using either a scalded blender jar or a scalded bowl with a hand blender or electric mixer. Add the remaining 2 cups of soymilk to the blended mixture, stirring with a scalded metal spoon or blending briefly in a blender or mixer. Try to avoid too many bubbles; you can cover the mixture tightly and allow it to sit in the refrigerator for a little while to dissipate the bubbles if necessary.

Pour the mixture into two sterilized pint canning jars. Bring the mixture to 110°F, either by placing the jars in a pan of hot water and heating them over medium-high heat, or by heating each jar in the microwave for about 40 seconds. Check the temperature with a sterilized thermometer. Whisk 1 tablespoon of the yogurt into each jar with a sterilized whisk. Cover the jars with sterilized lids, and place them in a foam cooler or ice chest with a covered jar of hot tap water. Cover the cooler and let sit for about 4 hours, or until the yogurt is firmly set. Check after 2 hours and at hourly intervals after that. It may take as long as 6 hours, but mine usually takes 4. When the yogurt is firm, place it in the refrigerator, where it will keep about 2 weeks.

Soy Buttermilk

You can make soy buttermilk in almost the same way as Thick Homemade Soy Yogurt, but omit the soy protein isolate powder and yogurt culture, and use about ½ cup of dairy buttermilk or a packaged buttermilk culture. (Follow the directions on the package for packaged culture). Instead of placing the jars in a cooler, simply keep them at room temperature. At 80°F, they thicken in as little as 2 hours. Use Soy Buttermilk as a beverage or in baking.

For baking, you can use soy yogurt, diluted with a little plain soymilk, in place of buttermilk. Or you can simply curdle 1 cup of soymilk with 1 tablespoon of lemon juice. I use these substitutions instead of beaten egg for coating vegetarian cutlets and vegetables before breading them for frying or baking.

Soy Yogurt Cheese

This tangy, creamy cheese can be made the same way as dairy yogurt cheese. Follow the directions for thick homemade soy yogurt. If you don't have a special yogurt cheese maker, drain the yogurt in a coffee filter or a couple of layers of fine mesh cheesecloth in a mesh strainer over a bowl. Cover and let the mixture drain in the refrigerator for 24 hours. The cheese can be salted to taste and used as you would use dairy yogurt cheese or cream cheese. You can add herbs if you wish. Remove the drained cheese to a covered container, and store in the refrigerator for up to 2 weeks.

Tofu-Fruit Yogurt

Yield: 4 servings

If you do not care for soy yogurt, or it is not available in your area, try this easy recipe instead; it has less of a soy flavor.

Per serving: Calories 89, Protein 6 g, Soy Protein 6 g, Fat 3 g, Carbohydrates 10 g

3 cups fresh or frozen berries, or other
   chunked fruit

One 12.3-ounce box firm or extra-firm
   silken tofu, crumbled

2¼ teaspoons vanilla

2 tablespoons fresh lemon juice

Pinch of salt

1 teaspoon nondairy acidophilus powder
   (optional)

Unbleached sugar or grade A light maple
   syrup to taste

Chop the berries or fruit in a blender or food processor. Add the crumbled tofu and continue blending. Add the vanilla, lemon juice, and salt. The resulting consistency should be similar to that of yogurt. Stir in the acidophilus powder if you want the benefits of this active culture, then chill the mixture until it firms up.

Sweeten each serving to taste with unbleached sugar or grade A light maple syrup.

Chai

Chai (spiced Indian tea), which is sold by street vendors all over India and Nepal, is all the rage as the alternative to espresso. You can buy mixes and even ready-made varieties in cartons. But it's very easy to make it at home. Be sure to use the cardamom in this recipe, but you can vary the other spices. Some possibilities are fennel, nutmeg, white peppercorns, star anise, allspice, coriander seeds, and vanilla. Tea has far less caffeine in it than coffee, but you can use a naturally decaffeinated variety if you can find an acceptable one, or use the herbal alternative suggested below.

Per serving: Calories 47, Protein 2 g, Soy Protein 2 g, Fat 1 g, Carbohydrates 7 g

3 cups water

4 whole cloves

1 teaspoon cardamom seeds

5 black peppercorns

1 stick cinnamon

1 quarter-size slice fresh ginger

¼ teaspoon anise seed

2 tablespoons loose black tea

1 to 1½ cups soymilk

About 2 tablespoons unbleached sugar, or to taste

Bring the water to a boil, and add the spices. Cover and simmer gently for 10 to 15 minutes. Turn off the heat and add the black tea. Cover and let steep for a few minutes. Heat the soymilk gently in a large saucepan. Strain the tea into the hot soymilk, and sweeten to taste. Serve hot.

❧ *Iced Chai:* Sweeten a little more than for hot tea, let it cool, and pour it over a tall glass of crushed ice.

❧ *Caffeine-Free Chai:* Omit the black tea and use Rooibos tea instead (2 bags if you can't find it loose). Rooibos (pronounced roy-bush; it means "red bush" in Afrikaans) is the bark of a bush in South African. This delicious herb tea is very popular there. We have been familiar with this tea for many years, because my husband has South African family connections and they send it to us, but it is just beginning to be known in North America. It has a slightly malty flavor and is the only herbal tea I know that can be enjoyed the way we Westerners prefer black tea—with milk and sugar. It reputedly has a high mineral content.

Chapter 8

Condiments, sauces, dips, dressings, and spreads

It's easy to slip soyfoods, especially tofu, into a wide variety of sauces and spreads. In this chapter you'll find familiar sauces, dips, and spreads that are creamy and rich-tasting, but I've converted them to be dairy-free and soy-rich; salad dressings are tangy and smooth. This group of recipes probably has more possibilities for fooling—and converting—soyphobes than any other. Most of these recipes are much lower in fat and calories than their dairy counterparts.

Tofu Mayonnaise

Yield: a generous 1½ cups

Silken tofu makes a smooth, thick, rich-tasting mayonnaise that doesn't separate. I think it tastes quite rich enough as it is, but if you like, you can add a little extra-virgin olive oil.

Per 2 tablespoons: Calories 18, Protein 2 g, Soy Protein 2 g, Fat 1 g,
Carbohydrates 1 g

One 12.3-ounce package extra-firm silken tofu

2 tablespoons cider vinegar or lemon juice

1⅛ teaspoons salt

½ teaspoon dry mustard

⅛ teaspoon white pepper

1 to 2 tablespoons extra-virgin olive oil (optional)

1 teaspoon sweetener (optional)

Combine the ingredients in a food processor or blender, and process until very smooth. Pour into a clean jar, close tightly, and refrigerate. This will keep for about 2 weeks in the refrigerator.

Soy Mayonnaise Makes about 2 cups

For those who do not like tofu mayonnaise or the commercial light mayos (most are not vegan, anyway), here is a delicious solution. It contains a small amount of oil, but a tablespoon of this mayo has only about 2 grams of fat, compared to 5 grams in light mayonnaise and 11 grams in regular.

Per 2 tablespoons: Calories 41, Protein 0 g, Soy Protein 0 g, Fat 3 g, Carbohydrates 2 g

½ cup + 2 tablespoons cold water

¾ teaspoon agar powder, or ½ tablespoon agar flakes

3 tablespoons cornstarch or wheat starch

1 cup soymilk

3 tablespoons apple cider or white wine vinegar

1½ teaspoons salt

¾ teaspoon dry mustard

Pinch white pepper or lemon pepper, to taste

¼ cup extra-virgin olive oil

Microwave Option:
In a microwave-proof bowl, pour the water over the agar, and stir in the cornstarch. Microwave on high for 30 seconds; whisk. Repeat three times, or until thick and translucent, not white. Follow the remaining instructions below.

You can use either Tofu Mayonnaise or Soy Mayonnaise for any of the variations below.

In a small saucepan, pour the water over the agar, and stir in cornstarch. Heat over high heat, stirring constantly, until thick and translucent, not white.

Remove the cornstarch mixture from the heat, and pour into a blender or food processor. Add all the remaining ingredients, except the oil, and blend well. While the machine is running, add the oil slowly through the top. Blend until the mixture is very white, frothy, and emulsified (you can't see any oil globules). Pour into a clean jar, cover, and refrigerate. It keeps for several weeks.

❧ *Aioli:* To make a delicious garlic dip for cold, steamed vegetables and artichokes, omit the dry mustard and add 4 to 6 peeled cloves of garlic while blending. This also makes a good spread for garlic toast.

❧ *Tartar Sauce:* After the mayonnaise has firmed up in the refrigerator, add ¾ cup minced raw onion and ¾ cup minced dill pickle. Add pickle brine to taste, if you wish. If you have no pickles, use chopped cucumber with dill and white wine vinegar to taste.

❧ *Russian Dressing:* Combine 1 cup of either mayonnaise, 1 tablespoon prepared horseradish, 1 teaspoon vegetarian Worcestershire sauce, ¼ cup ketchup-style chili sauce, and 1 teaspoon grated onion.

Flavored Mayonnaise

Flavored mayonnaise can turn quick sandwich or salad meals into a gourmet treat. Try these suggestions, then invent your own. Add any of the following to Tofu Mayonnaise (page 90), Soy Mayonnaise (page 89), or your favorite commercial mayonnaise. Or try them with Tofu-Cashew Cream Cheese (page 94).

- 3 tablespoons minced pickled jalapeños

- 3 minced chipotle chilis

- Several tablespoons of Vegan Pesto Genovese (page 105), puréed roasted red pepper, puréed soaked sun-dried tomato, or mashed roasted garlic

> *Bright Idea:* Tofu Mayonnaise and its variations can be used as savory vegetable and toast toppings. If you leave out the agar, they make good bases for cold savory sauces.

- 1 tablespoon minced or grated fresh ginger

- 2 tablespoons prepared horseradish

- 1 tablespoon curry powder

- ¼ cup or more minced fresh herbs, such as basil, mint, oregano, cilantro, and tarragon

- ⅓ cup chopped chives, 1 tablespoon grated lemon zest (preferably organic), and Louisiana hot sauce to taste

- 1 tablespoon Chinese hoisin sauce or ½ tablespoon each dark or red miso and maple syrup

- ¼ to ½ cup salsa

- 1 to 2 teaspoons wasabi powder (Japanese green horseradish)

- 2 tablespoons citrus zest, preferably organic

- ¼ to ⅓ cup minced Japanese-style pink pickled ginger

- 3 to 6 tablespoons of your favorite chutney

- 12 to 18 cloves (1 head) roasted garlic

- Use cranberry or other berry vinegar, balsamic or sherry vinegar, or lime juice instead of ordinary vinegar or lemon juice.

- Use your favorite herbal vinegar plus 3 to 4 tablespoons of minced fresh herbs.

- For a tasty sandwich spread, mix together one part Tofu Mayonnaise or Soy Mayonnaise and one part Dijon mustard (for a dijonnaise) or light miso.

Quick Tofu Ricotta Cheese

Yield: 1 generous cup

Per ¼ cup: Calories 47, Protein 4 g, Soy Protein 4 g, Fat 3 g, Carbohydrates 1 g

½ pound medium-firm tofu, mashed and drained

3 tablespoons soymilk

¼ teaspoon salt

Mix all the ingredients together in a bowl, and refrigerate.

Tofu Cottage Cheese

Yield: about 2½ cups

This is delicious with chives and/or chopped vegetables, or pineapple tidbits.

Per ¼ cup: Calories 47, Protein 4 g, Soy Protein 4 g, Fat 2 g, Carbohydrates 1 g

¾ teaspoon salt

1 pound medium-firm tofu, mashed coarsely and drained

⅔ cup firm or extra-firm silken tofu

1 tablespoon lemon juice

¼ teaspoon sugar or other sweetener

In a medium bowl, sprinkle ½ teaspoon of the salt on the mashed tofu. In a food processor, mix the silken tofu, remaining salt, lemon juice, and sugar until very smooth. Add to the mashed tofu, and mix gently. Refrigerate.

Tofu-Cashew Cream Cheese

Yield: 1 cup

This is a welcome and tasty innovation, cheaper and lower in fat than commercial nondairy cream cheese. And some brands contain casein, a dairy protein. Two tablespoons of regular dairy cream cheese contains about 10 grams of fat, and Tofutti Better Than Cream Cheese contains 8 grams.

Tofu-Cashew Cream Cheese, on the other hand, contains about 4 grams of fat per 2 tablespoons! It is rich-tasting, creamy-smooth, and delicious, and can be whipped up in minutes in your food processor. You can add fruit and spices for delicious variations. If you can't use a food processor for this recipe, combine all the ingredients in a bowl first, and process in small batches in a blender.

Per tablespoon: Calories 31, Protein 2 g, Soy Protein 1 g, Fat 2 g, Carbohydrates 2 g

One 12.3-ounce box extra-firm silken tofu, drained

⅓ cup raw cashew pieces, finely ground

5 teaspoons lemon juice

½ teaspoon salt

1 teaspoon sweetener of choice (optional)

Savory Gourmet Tofu Cream Cheese Spreads

Use any of the Flavored Mayonnaise variations (pages 92-93) with the Tofu-Cashew Cream Cheese Spread and Tofu-Miso Goat Cheese-Style Spread recipes on the facing page to make gourmet spreads. Also try mixing one recipe with ½ cup of your favorite chutney for a spicy cracker spread. Pesto (page 105), chopped sun-dried tomatoes, olives, and roasted peppers all make great flavorings.

Place the tofu in a clean tea towel, gather the ends together, and twist and squeeze for a couple of minutes to extract most of the water. Place all the ingredients in a food processor, and process for several minutes or until the mixture is very smooth. You may have to stop the machine and scrape the sides with a spatula once or twice. Use immediately or place in a covered container and refrigerate. (It firms up with refrigeration and will keep about 1 week.)

❧ *Italian-Style Tofu Ricotta* (makes about 1¾ cups): Do not squeeze the silken tofu. Use 3½ teaspoons lemon juice and ¼ teaspoon salt. Process about three-quarters of the tofu in a food processor, along with the ground cashews, lemon juice, and salt, until they are very smooth. Then crumble in the remaining tofu, and process again briefly. The resulting mixture should be mostly smooth but with a little graininess. Scoop into a container, cover, and refrigerate. It firms up when chilled.

❧ *Sweet Ricotta Cream:* This is delicious over fruit and other desserts. Blend one recipe of Italian-Style Tofu Ricotta (above) with ¼ cup grade A light maple syrup and 1 teaspoon vanilla until very smooth.

❧ *Tofu Devonshire Cream* (makes about 1⅓ cups): Use this on scones and other breads, or as a thick whipped cream substitute. Make the Tofu-Cashew Cream Cheese, but don't squeeze the tofu. Use only ¼ teaspoon salt, and add about 1½ tablespoons grade A maple syrup.

❧ *Tofu-Miso Goat Cheese-Style Spread* (makes 1 cup): Make the basic recipe but use only 2½ teaspoons of lemon juice and leave out the salt and optional sweetener. Add 2 tablespoons plus 1 teaspoon light miso. You may also add fresh or dried herbs, drained sun-dried tomatoes in oil, roasted peppers, garlic, etc.

❧ *Tofu-Cashew Sour Cream* (makes about 1¾ cups): This is richer than Tofu Sour Cream (page 97) but still has only about 2 grams of fat per tablespoon. Follow the directions for Tofu-Cashew Cream Cheese, but don't squeeze the tofu. Use 2 tablespoons plus 1 teaspoon lemon juice, and add ⅓ cup soymilk. Blend until very smooth and refrigerate.

❧ *Tofu Cream Cheese-Peanut Butter Spread* (makes about 1½ cups): If you crave peanut butter but want to cut the calories in half, try this. Make the Tofu-Cashew Cream Cheese, but omit the cashews and add ½ cup peanut butter, smooth or chunky, instead.

Nondairy Bechamel

Yield: 2 cups

I think this recipe is a great improvement upon vegan white sauces made completely with soymilk, which I find too sweet. The tofu and broth cube add richness without much fat. This rich-tasting sauce, used frequently in Italian cooking, is actually quite low in fat. It is a key ingredient in dishes such as lasagne. It can be used as an all-purpose white sauce in all of your cooking, and as a topping for Greek dishes, such as vegetarian moussaka.

Per ¼ cup: Calories 53, Protein 2 g, Soy Protein 2 g, Fat4 g, Carbohydrates 3 g

1 cup soymilk

½ cup crumbled extra-firm silken tofu or medium-firm regular tofu

½ cup water

1 chicken-style vegetarian broth cube, crumbled, or enough broth powder to flavor 1 cup liquid

½ teaspoon salt

2 tablespoons nondairy margarine or extra-virgin olive oil

1½ to 3 tablespoons unbleached flour

Large pinch each of freshly grated nutmeg and white pepper

To make this sauce wheat- and corn-free, melt the margarine and add it to the soymilk mixture, along with 1 to 4 tablespoons of white rice flour or mochiko flour, also known as sweet or glutinous rice flour, instead of the wheat flour. In other words, you don't need to make a cooked roux. Four tablespoons of flour makes a very thick sauce. Sauces made with mochiko flour are excellent for freezing (for instance, in a prepared but not baked lasagne), because the sauce will not separate when thawed.

Place the soymilk, tofu, water, broth cube or powder, and salt in a blender, and mix until very smooth. Set aside.

In a medium, heavy saucepan over medium-high heat, melt the margarine and whisk in 1½ tablespoons of flour, adding more if necessary to make the mixture thicker. Whisk for a few minutes, but remove from the heat just before it starts to change color. (You want a white roux.) Add to the soymilk mixture in the blender, and process for a few seconds. Pour the mixture back into the saucepan. Cook over medium-high heat, stirring frequently, until the sauce thickens and boils. Reduce the temperature to low, and simmer for a few minutes to cook thoroughly. Whisk in the nutmeg and pepper.

Microwave Option: Using a large microwave-safe bowl, melt the margarine in the microwave on high for 45 seconds. Whisk in the flour and microwave on high for 2 minutes. Add to the soymilk mixture in the blender, and process briefly, then pour the mixture back into the bowl. Microwave on high for 2 minutes. Whisk. Microwave for 2 more minutes, then whisk again. Microwave for 2 minutes more, and whisk in the nutmeg and pepper.

Tofu Sour Cream or Yogurt

Yield: 1½ cups

Silken tofu makes a smooth, rich-tasting cream that can be used any time you would normally use sour cream. You can even cook with it. For a slightly richer sour cream, see the variation of Tofu Cream Cheese Spread called Tofu-Cashew Sour Cream (page 95).

Per ¼ cup: Calories 39, Protein 4 g, Soy Protein 4 g, Fat 2 g, Carbohydrates 2 g

One 12.3-ounce package extra-firm silken tofu

3 tablespoons lemon juice

½ teaspoon unbleached sugar

¼ teaspoon salt

Process all the ingredients in a food processor or blender until very smooth. This will keep in a covered container in the refrigerator for up to a week.

♪ *Creamy Fruit Topping:* Sweeten the sour cream with a tablespoon or two of grade A light maple syrup, fruit-sweetened jam or jelly, fruit juice concentrate, or fruit liqueur.

♪ *Tofu Yogurt:* There are several brands of soy yogurt now available in natural food stores, but I prefer this for sauces and cooking. Reduce the salt to a small pinch, and increase the lemon juice to 4 tablespoons. If the cream seems too thick, thin it with some water to make it the consistency you prefer.

Cheddary Spread

Yield: about 1¼ cups

This variation of Crock Cheese from The Nutritional Yeast Cookbook by Joanne Stepaniak makes a very tangy spread, great on crackers or in celery sticks.

Per 2 tablespoons: Calories 53, Protein 4 g, Soy Protein 2 g, Fat 3 g, Carbohydrates 4 g

One 12.3-ounce box extra-firm silken tofu, drained

2 tablespoons sesame tahini

2 tablespoons lemon juice

¾ teaspoon salt

1 teaspoon sweetener of choice (optional)

¼ cup nutritional yeast flakes

1½ tablespoons light miso

1 teaspoon onion powder

1 teaspoon paprika

¼ teaspoon garlic granules

¼ teaspoon tumeric

¼ teaspoon dry mustard

Place the tofu in a clean tea towel, gather the ends together, and twist and squeeze for a couple of minutes to extract most of the water. Place all the ingredients in a food processor, and process for several minutes or until the mixture is very smooth. You may have to stop the machine and scrape the sides with a spatula once or twice. Use immediately or place in a covered container. and refrigerate.

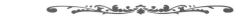

Tofu Herb Sauce

Yield: 1 cup

Per 2 tablespoons: Calories 17, Protein 2 g, Soy Protein 2 g, Fat 1 g, Carbohydrates 1 g

⅔ cup firm or extra-firm silken tofu

¼ cup lemon juice

2 cloves garlic

1 teaspoon dried mint, 1 tablespoon chopped fresh mint, or ¼ cup chopped fresh parsley

½ teaspoon salt

Pinch of sugar

Pepper, to taste

2 tablespoons tahini (optional)

Bright Idea: This is especially good on the Soyfelafel, page 124.

Combine all the ingredients in a food processor or blender, and process until very smooth.

Tofu Mascarpone

Yield: about 2 cups

Mascarpone is a very rich triple-cream cheese, mild and a bit more yellow than cream. It is often used as a substitute for whipped cream on Italian desserts. In North America, ordinary cream cheese is often used instead. If you can obtain it, Tofutti's "Better Than Cream Cheese" also makes a good substitute. Otherwise, try this easy version.

Per tablespoon: Calories 24, Protein 1 g, Soy Protein 1 g, Fat 2 g, Carbohydrates 1 g

One 12.3-ounce package extra-firm silken tofu

½ cup plus 2 tablespoons raw cashew pieces, very finely ground

6 teaspoons fresh lemon juice

Pinch of salt

Process all of the ingredients in a food processor or blender at high speed for several minutes. Be patient; it has to be very smooth. You may have to stop the machine a couple of times and scrape down the sides. When the mixture is as smooth as possible, scoop into a covered container, and refrigerate for up to 1 week. It will firm up considerably.

Easy Soy Cream for Cooking

When you need some heavy cream—say, as a binding in ravioli filling, for creamy soup, or as a thickener for vegetable pasta sauce—make sure you have some soymilk and a box of extra-firm silken tofu on hand. Just process an equal amount of soymilk and silken tofu in a blender or food processor until it is very smooth, and add it to your recipe. (You can even use a miniprocessor or a hand blender for small amounts.) With this formula, you don't have to make up a whole recipe ahead of time and perhaps have half of it hanging around in the fridge waiting to be used.

For instance, if you need ½ cup cream for your recipe, blend ¼ cup soymilk with ¼ cup extra-firm silken tofu.

Don't worry about seasoning it, because you can further season the food you are adding it to.

Pourable Nondairy Cream

Yield: 1 cup

You determine the thickness of this rich-tasting nondairy cream by which type of silken tofu you use. Choose soft for cream to pour over cereal and firm or extra-firm for a thicker pouring cream. For a cream that has no discernible soy flavor, blend the tofu with a mild-tasting nondairy milk.

Per ¼ cup: Calories 39, Protein 2 g, Soy Protein 2 g, Fat 1 g, Carbohydrates 5 g

½ cup crumbled silken tofu

½ cup nondairy milk, such as almond or rice

4 teaspoons grade A light maple syrup

⅛ teaspoon coconut extract*

Pinch of salt

*The coconut extract doesn't make the cream taste like coconut but gives it a rich flavor.

Place all the ingredients in a blender or food processor, and process until very smooth. Pour into a covered container, and refrigerate for several hours, or overnight, before using. It will keep about 4 days.

Chips and Dippers

Besides raw vegetable dippers, or crudités, there are now some wonderful baked tortilla and potato chips available from natural food stores and supermarkets, which have little or no fat. From your supermarket you can buy pita crisps and bagel chips, melba toast, rye crisp bread, fat-free crackers, brown rice wafers, rice cakes, baked pretzels, and bread sticks (crispini). Check the ingredients and fat content on the labels before buying; they vary from brand to brand.

Vegetable Dip

Don't use a soup mix that contains potatoes in this dip, or the results will be too thick and gloppy.

Per 2 tablespoons: Calories 26, Protein 2 g, Soy Protein 2 g, Fat 1 g, Carbohydrates 2 g

1⅓ cups extra-firm silken tofu

2 tablespoons lemon juice

One ¾-ounce package vegetable soup mix

¼ teaspoon salt

Mix all the ingredients in a food processor or blender, and process until smooth. Place in a bowl, cover, and refrigerate. Serve with crackers, low-fat baked potato chips, or raw vegetables.

❧ *Onion Dip:* Substitute ¾ ounce of vegetarian onion soup mix for the vegetable soup mix.

Quick, Simple Soy Dips

Start with Tofu Sour Cream (page 97), Tofu-Cashew Cream Cheese (page 94), Soy Mayonnaise (page 91), Tofu Mayonnaise (page 90), or puréed cooked or canned green soybeans. Flavor simply with herbal salt or seasoned salt, or pesto (page 105) to taste. Or add ½ cup puréed roasted red peppers (from a jar), or puréed reconstituted dried tomatoes or sun-dried tomatoes in oil. Add some chopped fresh garlic, maybe a chopped green onion or two or some chives, and some chopped fresh herbs. Add a little more lemon juice if you like.

Or just add lots of fresh herbs, such as dill and basil, with a little more salt and lemon juice to taste.

For a Mexican-style dip, add your favorite hot tomato salsa to taste, and serve with baked tortilla chips.

Tofu-Soy Parmesan Spread

Yield: about 2 cups

This is delicious on crostini or crackers. Vary it by adding other herbs, chopped and drained oil-packed sun-dried tomatoes, roasted red peppers, marinated artichokes, kalamata olives, or toasted pine nuts, almonds, or other nuts.

Per 2 tablespoons: Calories 30, Protein 4 g, Soy Protein 4 g, Fat 2 g, Carbohydrates 1 g

⅓ cup fresh basil, packed

1 large clove garlic, peeled

One 12.3-ounce package extra-firm silken tofu

2 tablespoons fresh lemon juice

¾ teaspoon salt

Pinch of white pepper

¾ cup soy Parmesan

Mince the basil and garlic finely in a food processor. Add the tofu, lemon juice, salt, and pepper. Process until smooth. Add the soy Parmesan and process again until smooth. Pour into a serving bowl, cover, and chill until serving time.

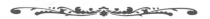

Miso Caesar Dressing

Yield: about 1¼ cups

Here miso takes the place of anchovies. Toss the dressing with crisp Romaine lettuce, croutons, and some soy Parmesan to taste. This makes enough for two company-size salads.

Per 2 tablespoons: Calories 20, Protein 1 g, Soy Protein 1 g, Fat 1 g, Carbohydrates 2 g

⅔ cup medium-firm regular tofu or firm or extra-firm silken tofu

¼ cup water, vegetable broth, or broth from cooking beans

¼ cup fresh lemon juice

2 tablespoons light miso

1 tablespoon red wine vinegar

1 teaspoon Dijon mustard

2 cloves garlic, peeled

½ teaspoon each salt and pepper

2 dashes of Louisiana hot sauce

¼ teaspoon vegetarian Worcestershire sauce (optional)

Process all the ingredients in a blender until smooth.

Melty Soy Pizza Cheese

This easy recipe is tastier than any commercial vegan cheese substitute—and much cheaper. Drizzle it hot over pizza or casseroles before baking. I think it's most appealing if you also run it briefly under the broiler after baking, just enough to make it really bubbly, with a thin crust on top. If you want to use it on cold sandwiches, spread the cooled mixture onto the bread. The optional calcium carbonate powder (available from your pharmacy) gives 2 tablespoons of the cheese about the same amount of calcium as 1 ounce of dairy cheese, and the nutritional yeast adds protein and lots of B-complex vitamins, as well as cheesy flavor.

Per ¼ cup: Calories 96, Protein 7 g, Soy Protein 3 g, Fat 5 g, Carbohydrates 7 g

1 cup soymilk

¼ cup nutritional yeast flakes

2 tablespoons cornstarch

1 tablespoon white flour

2 tablespoons soy protein isolate powder

1 teaspoon lemon juice

½ teaspoon salt

¼ teaspoon garlic granules

4 teaspoons calcium carbonate powder (optional)

2 tablespoons water

1 to 2 tablespoons canola oil or other neutral-tasting vegetable oil

Place the soymilk, yeast, cornstarch, flour, soy protein isolate powder, lemon juice, salt, garlic granules, and calcium, if using, in a blender, and process until smooth. Pour the mixture into a small saucepan. Stir over medium heat until it starts to thicken, then let bubble 30 seconds and whisk vigorously.

Microwave Option: Pour the mixture into a medium microwave-proof bowl. Microwave on high for 2 minutes, whisk, then microwave at 50 percent (or medium) power for 2 minutes, and whisk again.

Whisk in the water and oil. Drizzle immediately over pizza or other food, and bake or broil until a skin forms on top. Or refrigerate for up to a week. It will get quite firm upon chilling but will still be spreadable. You can spread the firm cheese on bread or quesadillas for grilling, or heat to thin it out for pouring over food. Refrigerated, this keeps for about one week.

Rich Brown Yeast Gravy

Yield: about 2½ cups

This fat-free and delicious brown gravy is one of my favorite staples. It can be made ahead and reheated.

Per ¼ cup: Calories 27, Protein 3 g, Soy Protein 0 g, Fat 0 g, Carbohydrates 4 g

⅓ cup nutritional yeast flakes

⅓ cup unbleached white flour

2½ cups water

2 tablespoons soy sauce

½ teaspoon salt

A few shakes of Kitchen Bouquet or other gravy browner, or mushroom soy sauce, which is darker (optional)

Bright Idea: For a giblet-style gravy, add about 1 cup of chopped reconstituted textured soy protein chunks (page 54) or sautéed mushrooms before cooking.

In a heavy saucepan over high heat, whisk the yeast and flour together for a minute until it smells toasted. Remove from the heat and whisk in the water, soy sauce, salt, and Kitchen Bouquet, if desired. Cook over high heat, stirring constantly, until the mixture thickens and comes to a boil. Reduce the heat and simmer on low for 4 to 5 minutes.

Microwave Option: In a 1½-quart microwave-proof bowl, mix the yeast and flour. Cook uncovered in the microwave on high for 3 minutes. Whisk in the remaining ingredients, cover, and cook on high for 3 minutes. Whisk again, cover, and cook on high again for 3 minutes. Whisk.

You also can make half the recipe in a 4-cup microwave-safe glass measuring container. Cook as above, but in 2-minute increments.

Vegan Pesto Genovese

Yield: about 1½ cups

To serve pesto with pasta, dilute it with a little of the pasta cooking water before tossing with the pasta.

Per tablespoon: Calories 53, Protein 1 g, Soy Protein 1 g, Fat 6 g, Carbohydrates 0 g

4 cups packed fresh basil leaves

⅓ cup soy Parmesan

½ cup extra-virgin olive oil

¼ cup lightly toasted pine nuts, chopped walnuts, hazelnuts, almonds, or Brazil nuts

2 to 4 cloves garlic

1 teaspoon salt

½ tablespoon lemon juice (optional; to preserve the color)

Place all the ingredients in a food processor or in several batches in a blender, and process until the mixture forms a paste. Place the mixture in 2 or 3 small containers; the less air the pesto is exposed to, the better its color will be preserved. Cover the pesto with a thin film of olive oil or a piece of plastic wrap touching the pesto, to prevent discoloration, and cover tightly. Refrigerate. Use within 2 or 3 days. Otherwise, freeze the pesto in small containers or ice cube trays; don't freeze for more than a month or so, because it loses flavor.

❧ *Low-Fat Pesto:* Omit all or some of the oil, and substitute an equal amount of medium-firm or silken tofu.

❧ *Winter Pesto:* This is an authentic method of stretching expensive store-bought fresh basil during the winter months. Use 2 cups packed fresh basil leaves and 2 cups packed fresh Italian parsley leaves, and add about 2 tablespoons of chopped fresh marjoram if you can find it.

❧ *Pesto-Filled Mushrooms:* For a wonderful appetizer, spread pesto in large, stemmed mushroom caps, and broil about 3 to 4 inches from a heat source until the mushrooms are tender and juicy.

Quick Tofu Feta

Yield: about 1½ cups

This is excellent and very easy to make, especially in a microwave. It even melts when heated, so you can grill the chèvre variation in grape leaves or coat it in bread crumbs and fry until crispy on the outside and soft in the middle. This versatile recipe will allow you to easily convert many ethnic recipes to make them low-fat, nondairy, and soy-rich.

Per ¼ cup: Calories 48, Protein 2 g, Soy Protein 2 g, Fat 3 g, Carbohydrates 2 g

¾ cup crumbled firm tofu

1 teaspoon agar powder, or 2 tablespoons agar flakes

2 tablespoons water

½ teaspoon unbleached sugar

1 tablespoon canola oil

1¼ teaspoons salt

½ tablespoon light miso

3 tablespoons fresh lemon juice

Process the tofu, agar, water, sugar, oil, and salt in a food processor or blender until very smooth. Place the mixture in a small, heavy-bottomed saucepan. Cook over medium heat, stirring constantly, until it bubbles for a few minutes and thickens.

Microwave Option: Place the mixture in a microwave-safe bowl and microwave on high for 2 minutes. Whisk briefly. Microwave 1 minute more.

Whisk the miso and lemon juice into the cooked mixture.

Pour the mixture into a flat container, cover, and chill until firm. Cut into squares. You can refrigerate the squares in a jar, covered to the top in canola oil, up to several weeks. Rinse the oil off before using. Avoid storing in olive oil, which may thicken with refrigeration.

❧ *Ricotta Salata* (a salty dry ricotta that can be crumbled or grated and is used in some Italian recipes and on pastas): Use only 1 teaspoon salt. This can be stored in oil like Quick Tofu Feta (see above). This also makes a good Mexican Queso Fresco (ubiquitous mild fresh Mexican white cheese)

❧ *Creamy Version:* Instead of firm tofu, use 1⅓ cups extra-firm silken tofu and increase the amount of agar to 1½ teaspoons powder or 2½ tablespoons flakes.

♣ *Chèvre* (creamy goat cheese): Use 1⅓ cups extra-firm silken tofu, 1½ teaspoons agar powder (2½ tablespoons flakes), 2 tablespoons tahini, 2 tablespoons water, ½ teaspoon salt, 2 tablespoons miso, and 4 teaspoons lemon juice. You can roll this into balls or logs when almost firm, roll in peppercorns or herbs, and then store in the refrigerator in a jar of canola oil to cover.

♣ *Yogurt Cheese* and *Yogurt Cheese Balls* (used in Middle Eastern cooking): Use the Creamy Version but use only ¾ teaspoon salt and omit the miso. Good for spreading on pita crisps, rye crisp, and sesame crackers. Or after refrigerating until firm, roll the cheese into balls and store in a jar of oil in the refrigerator. You can roll the balls in herbs (thyme is especially good), zatar (a sumac-thyme-sesame mixture), or Aleppo pepper before you add them to the jar of oil. Or add bay leaves, thyme sprigs, and red chiles to the jar.

Mushroom-Tofu Pâté

Yield: 4 to 6 servings (1⅓ cups)

This is so easy and very delicious. It firms up enough to unmold and is always a hit at parties and potlucks. (You can easily double the recipe.)

Per serving: Calories 45, Protein 3 g, Soy Protein 3 g, Fat 1 g, Carbohydrates 4 g

⅓ cup dried boletus or porcini mushrooms, or ½ cup coarsely crumbled stemmed dried shiitake or Chinese mushrooms

¾ cup crumbled firm tofu

2 tablespoons light miso

2 to 3 large fresh basil leaves or ½ teaspoon dried basil

1 head roasted garlic, with the pulp squeezed out of the skins, or 8 to 12 cloves commercial roasted garlic from a jar

¼ teaspoon salt

1 to 2 tablespoons extra-virgin olive oil (optional)

Soak the mushrooms for ½ hour in boiling water to cover. Drain them in a fine mesh strainer, and squeeze them dry. (Save the soaking water for soup or stock.) Chop the mushrooms in a food processor, then add the remaining ingredients and process until quite smooth. Pack the mixture into a small, oiled bowl, and chill at least 12 hours. When ready to serve, loosen the edges of the pâté with a knife, and turn it out onto a plate. Decorate with a sprig of fresh basil, and serve with crackers or crostini.

Guacamole

Yield: about 4 cups

Born and raised in California, I love avocadoes, but their high fat content makes them a rare treat. The following easy bean mixture, a variation of the one in my second cookbook, The Almost No-Fat Holiday Cookbook, *makes a very tasty alternative. (You need a food processor for this recipe.)*

Per ¼ cup: Calories 46, Protein 4 g, Soy Protein 3 g, Fat 1 g, Carbohydrates 4 g

10 ounces small, whole fresh or frozen green beans

10 ounces frozen sweet beans (green soybeans) or baby lima beans

1 cup medium-firm regular tofu or firm or extra-firm silken tofu

½ cup spicy tomato salsa

4 to 6 tablespoons lemon juice

4 cloves garlic, crushed

2 teaspoons salt

1 teaspoon ground cumin

1 ripe avocado, pitted and peeled (optional)

Cook the green beans and sweet beans separately, both in water just to cover, until tender and still bright green, but not mushy (approximately 5 minutes). Drain the beans and place in a food processor. Blend until smooth. Add the remaining ingredients and blend again until smooth. Place in a covered bowl, and refrigerate.

Marinated Tofu Cubes

This is an easy and delicious way to add tofu to your diet. Cut firm tofu into small cubes, and cover them in a jar with a light vinaigrette dressing, preferably low-fat. You can use a vinaigrette made with any sort of vinegar, but red wine or balsamic vinegar will turn the tofu a rosy color. Add sprigs of fresh herbs, whole dried chilies, and whole cloves of garlic to the jar if you like. If sealed tightly, the tofu cubes will keep for up to three weeks in the refrigerator. Shake the container every now and then.

Use the tofu cubes in salads, stir-fries, grilled kebabs, or even crumbled on pizza.

Hot Artichoke Dip

Yield: about 3½ cups

This easy hot dip never fails to please. Serve it with crackers, crostini, or French bread.

Per 2 tablespoons: Calories 32, Protein 1 g, Soy Protein 1 g, Fat 2 g,
Carbohydrates 2 g

One 12-ounce jar marinated artichoke
  hearts, drained

1 cup commercial or homemade Tofu
  Mayonnaise (page 90) or Soy Mayonnaise
  (page 91)

½ cup soy Parmesan

3 tablespoons chopped fresh tarragon,
  basil, or dill (optional)

1 or more cloves garlic, crushed

Preheat the oven to 350°F. Combine all the ingredients in a food processor or blender, or process until the artichokes are coarsely chopped.

Place in an oven-proof or microwave-proof serving bowl, and sprinkle with paprika. Bake for 10 minutes or microwave on high for 2 minutes.

Red Chili Paste

Yield: 1¾ cups

Per tablespoon: Calories 12, Protein 0 g, Soy Protein 0 g, Fat 1 g, Carbohydrates 1 g

½ cup good-quality chili powder

7 tablespoons red wine vinegar

2 tablespoons dried red chili
  pepper flakes

4 vegetarian broth cubes,
  crumbled, or enough broth
  powder to flavor 4 cups liquid

1 tablespoon water

1 tablespoon salt

1 tablespoon olive oil or toasted
  sesame oil

1 tablespoon flour or 2 teaspoons
  rice flour

1 tablespoon Marmite, other yeast
  extract, or dark miso

6 cloves garlic, peeled

½ teaspoon each dried oregano and
  ground cumin

Mix all the ingredients in a food processor or blender until smooth. Store in the refrigerator.

Chapter 9

Appetizers, salads, and soups

Soyfoods can make nondairy, low-fat soups and salad dressings creamy and rich-tasting, and add hearty soy protein to whole-meal salads.

Oven-Fried Tofu

Yields 8 pieces

Preheat the oven to 500°F. Cut a block of firm tofu in half lengthwise, so you have two long pieces. Then cut each piece in half. Then cut each piece into triangles, so you have 8 triangles. Place these on dark, oiled cookie sheets (which help foods brown better), and brush the triangles with vegetable oil. Bake for 5 to 7 minutes per side or until golden and puffy. These may be frozen for future use.

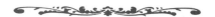

Edamamé (green soybeans in the pod)

This is a favorite snack in Japan, and it is addictive! The green soybeans are delicious and nutty tasting.

You should be able to find green soybeans frozen in the pod in Asian or Japanese markets.

Boil or steam the fresh or frozen pods of green soybeansfor about 20 minutes. Drain and serve them warm, allowing everyone to salt his or her own portion.

To eat edamamé, place a pod in your mouth, and close your teeth over the end, still holding onto the tip of the pod with your fingers. Pull the pod out of your mouth, with your teeth still closed, and the beans (and a little of the salt on the pod) will pop out into your mouth. Discard the pods and enjoy the tender little beans.

Soynuts

Soynuts are dry-roasted soybeans. They are delicious as a crunchy snack or can be used in some recipes in place of roasted seeds or nuts.

Soak dry soybeans overnight in enough water to cover generously. Drain, rinse, and place in a pot with enough fresh water to cover. Bring to a boil, then lower the heat and simmer for 10 minutes. Drain.

Preheat the oven to 350°F. Spread the beans in a single layer on lightly oiled cookie sheets. Roast them for about 45 minutes, or until golden and crispy, stirring several times while roasting. Cool thoroughly, then store in airtight containers. They can be frozen.

You can coat the roasted soybeans with a tiny bit of oil, using one of those new pump sprayers, if you have one. Then salt them, or add any number of flavorings, such as garlic granules, or Cajun or Indian spices.

Eggless Egg Salad Yield: 3 cups

This is delicious not only on sandwiches but also on crackers and celery sticks.

Per ¼ cup: Calories 60, Protein 4 g, Soy Protein 4 g, Fat 2 g, Carbohydrates 2 g

2½ cups medium-firm or firm tofu (1¼ pounds)

½ cup Soy Mayonnaise (page 91) or Tofu Mayonnaise (page 90)

2 green onions, chopped

1 stalk celery, minced

2 tablespoons nutritional yeast flakes

2 teaspoons dried dill

2 teaspoons turmeric

1½ teaspoons prepared mustard

1 clove garlic, crushed, or ¼ teaspoon garlic granules

Paprika, salt, and pepper, to taste

2 tablespoons minced dill pickle (optional)

½ small green or red pepper, seeded and chopped

Crumble the tofu into a bowl, and mash coarsely with a fork. Mix in the remaining ingredients, cover, and refrigerate.

Thai Tofu Salad

Yield: 6 servings

This makes a great hot-weather main dish all on its own. It's so easy to throw together and can be made ahead of time.

Per serving: Calories 276, Protein 15 g, Soy Protein 13 g, Fat 6 g, Carbohydrates 39 g

6 ounces rice vermicelli or thin rice noodles

2 pounds prepared Breast of Tofu (page 144) or a commercial savory marinated or baked tofu, cut into slivers

1 peeled cucumber, cut into thin strips about 2 to 3 inches long

1½ large red bell peppers, seeded and cut into thin strips

⅓ cup chopped fresh mint, basil, or cilantro

Dressing:

6 tablespoons light soy sauce

4½ tablespoons fresh lime juice

3 tablespoons unbleached sugar

1½ tablespoons minced fresh ginger

1½ tablespoons minced pickled jalapeño pepper

1 large clove garlic, crushed

In a large bowl, cover the rice vermicelli with boiling water. Let stand for 3 minutes, or until softened, then drain and rinse well. Combine the vermicelli in the bowl with the tofu, cucumber, bell pepper, and fresh herbs.

Whisk the dressing ingredients together, and pour over the salad. Toss well. Serve at room temperature on a platter decorated with fresh mint, basil, and/or cilantro.

Garlic Slaw

This will wake up a sleepy winter palate!

Per serving: Calories 58, Protein 2 g, Soy Protein 1 g, Fat 1 g,
Carbohydrates 11 g

Dressing:

⅞ cup soymilk

⅓ cup cider vinegar

¼ cup grade A light maple syrup

¼ cup firm silken tofu or medium-
  firm regular tofu

4 large cloves garlic, peeled

1 teaspoon salt

8 cups finely shredded or chopped
  green cabbage or a combination
  of cabbage and grated carrot

Combine the dressing ingredients in a blender until very smooth, then toss in a large bowl with the shredded cabbage or cabbage and carrots. Cover the bowl and refrigerate until serving time.

Pasta Primavera Salad

Yield: 6 to 8 servings

Here's a hearty full-meal salad that's good enough to serve to company. If you're allergic to wheat, use rice pasta instead.

Per serving: Calories 221, Protein 11 g, Soy Protein 3 g, Fat 2 g, Carbohydrates 40 g

Salad:

¾ pound uncooked rotelle or fusilli (corkscrew) pasta

2 medium carrots, peeled and cut into thin oval slices, or 3 cups frozen sliced carrots

½ pound frozen whole small green beans

1 large onion, chopped

One 15-ounce can white kidney (cannellini) beans or chick-peas, drained (1½ cups cooked)

1 green bell pepper, seeded and diced

1 red bell pepper, seeded and diced

1 cup thinly sliced celery

2 tablespoons white wine vinegar

1 teaspoon salt

Freshly ground black pepper, to taste

Dressing:

One 12.3-ounce package firm or extra-firm silken tofu

¼ cup lemon juice

¼ cup chopped fresh basil, or 1½ tablespoons dried basil

1 tablespoon white wine vinegar

1 teaspoon salt

½ teaspoon dry mustard powder

Cook the pasta according to package directions. When the pasta is almost half-cooked, add the raw carrots, if using, to the pot. When the pasta is almost tender, add the green beans and frozen carrot slices, if using. When the pasta is just tender but still chewy, drain it, with the carrots and green beans, in a colander.

Place the drained pasta and vegetables in a large serving bowl with the onion, beans, peppers, and celery. Add the remaining salad ingredients, and toss well.

Place the dressing ingredients in a blender or food processor, and process until very smooth. Pour the dressing over the warm pasta, and combine well. Cover and refrigerate until serving time. Serve cold or at room temperature.

Japanese Noodle Soup

Yield: 4 to 6 servings

This is an easy, inexpensive, and delicious meal for days when you have little time or energy.

Per serving: Calories 178, Protein 11 g, Soy Protein 5 g, Fat 3 g, Carbohydrates 21 g

4 cups water

4 cups vegetarian broth

¼ cup dry sherry

¼ cup Japanese soy sauce

1 teaspoon grated ginger

¾ pound firm tofu or Oven-Fried Tofu (page 110)

2 carrots, julienned

8 ounces noodles, such as soba or spaghettini, cooked and drained

2 cups snow peas, 1 cup frozen baby peas, or 1½ cups sliced mushrooms

One 10-ounce package cleaned fresh spinach, or 3 cups finely shredded cabbage or thinly sliced broccoli florets

Sliced green onions, for garnish

Toasted sesame oil, for garnish

Bring the water and broth to a boil in a large pot. Add the sherry, soy sauce, ginger, tofu, and carrots, and simmer for 5 minutes. Add the cooked noodles and cabbage, if using, and simmer for 2 minutes. Add the peas and spinach, if using, and simmer 1 more minute. Garnish each serving with green onions and a sprinkle of sesame oil.

Cheesy Corn and Frank Chowder

Yield: 6 servings

Vegetarian franks can have a life beyond the hot dog bun, as this delicious recipe will prove.

Per serving: Calories 237, Protein 15 g, Soy Protein 11 g, Fat 4 g, Carbohydrates 31 g

1 large onion, chopped

4 cloves garlic, minced

1 cup sliced celery

4 cups vegetarian broth

1 pound (4 medium) waxy potatoes, peeled or unpeeled and diced

1 cup frozen corn kernels

4 tofu or other vegetarian franks, thinly sliced into rounds

¼ cup nutritional yeast flakes

¼ cup minced fresh parsley

2 teaspoons dry mustard

1 teaspoon salt, or 1 tablespoon light miso plus ½ teaspoon salt

¼ teaspoon black or white pepper

1 pound medium-firm tofu

1½ tablespoons lemon juice

1 tablespoon cornstarch

In a medium pot, steam-fry (see page 67) the onion, garlic, and celery until they begin to soften, about 5 minutes. Add the broth, potatoes, and corn. Simmer about 10 minutes, or until the potatoes are soft. Stir in the frank slices, yeast, parsley, mustard, salt, and pepper.

Pour a few tablespoons of the broth into a blender. Add the tofu, cornstarch, and lemon juice, and purée until very smooth. Pour the tofu mixture into the broth pot, and stir over medium-high heat until it thickens. Serve immediately.

New England-Style
Sea Vegetable Chowder

Yield: 4 to 6 servings

Dulse is a sea vegetable that is gathered on the northeastern coast of North America, so I thought it would be an appropriate substitute for the clam flavor. For flavor and texture, this soup rivals calorie-rich and fat-laden versions.

Per serving: Calories 194, Protein 11 g, Soy Protein 9 g, Fat 2 g,
Carbohydrates 33 g

Vegetable Base:

1 large onion, chopped

4 medium (about 1 pound) waxy potatoes, peeled and diced

2 cups vegetarian broth

½ cup dry textured soy protein granules

½ cup water

1 cup frozen corn kernels

½ cup crumbled dry dulse, or ¼ cup dulse flakes

¼ cup minced fresh parsley

1 bay leaf

1 tablespoon soy bacon chips

½ teaspoon dried thyme

¼ teaspoon kelp powder

Tofu Mixture:

1 cup medium-firm regular tofu or extra-firm silken tofu

1 cup water

2 teaspoons salt

1 teaspoon sweetener

Freshly ground black pepper, to taste

Paprika

In a medium pot, steam-fry (see page 67) the onions for about 5 minutes, or until softened. Add all the vegetable base ingredients. Cover and simmer for about 10 minutes, or until the potatoes are soft.

Meanwhile, whip all the tofu mixture ingredients in a blender until very smooth.

When the potatoes are soft, stir in the tofu mixture, add pepper to taste, and heat gently. Sprinkle each serving with paprika, and serve with crackers.

Peruvian Corn Chowder

Yield: 8 to 10 servings

Peruvians love their chowders, also called "chupe," and my father was no exception. I know he would have loved this low-fat, low-cholesterol version. Dulse, by the way, is a purple sea vegetable. The flakes are available in natural food stores. This soup is traditionally made with yellow potatoes, so use Yukon Gold potatoes or another yellow variety if at all possible.

Per serving: Calories 255, Protein 6 g, Soy Protein 2 g, Fat 4 g, Carbohydrates 44 g

2 cups minced onion

2 large cloves garlic, minced

2 tablespoons extra-virgin olive oil

½ cup chopped fresh tomato or canned diced tomato

1 crushed dried red chile pepper

½ teaspoon dried oregano

¼ teaspoon freshly ground black pepper

8 cups vegetarian broth

2 large Yukon Gold potatoes, peeled and cut into 1-inch cubes

2 tablespoons dulse flakes

2 teaspoons unbleached sugar

1 teaspoon tumeric

1½ pounds Yukon Gold potatoes, peeled and cut lengthwise into wedges

½ cup basmati rice

1 cup frozen baby peas

2 cups fresh or frozen corn kernels

½ pound medium-firm tofu

½ cup dry white wine or nonalcoholic white wine

1 teaspoon salt, or to taste

Corn on the cob, cut into 2-inch chunks

Minced fresh parsley, for garnish

In a large soup pot, sauté the onion and garlic in the olive oil over medium heat until the onion is softened. Add the tomato, chile pepper, oregano, and black pepper. Sauté 3 more minutes. Add the broth, 2 cubed potatoes, dulse, sugar, tumeric, and kelp powder. Bring to a boil, then lower the heat, cover, and simmer for 20 minutes, or until the potatoes are tender. Strain the mixture through a colander, pouring the broth back into the pot. Place the solids in a blender or food processor with 1½ cups of the broth. Leave an opening in the lid or feeder tube, but cover it with a folded towel. (If you close the top of the machine, the hot steam can cause an explosion.) Purée until smooth.

Add the puréed mixture back into the broth. Add the potato wedges and rice. Cover and bring to a simmer, stirring well to make sure that the rice kernels don't stick to the bottom of the pot. Simmer 25 minutes, stirring occasionally. Add the peas and corn kernels, and simmer 10 minutes.

Combine the tofu, wine, and salt in a blender or food processor, and process until very smooth. Add to the pot and heat gently. Add salt to taste.

To serve the traditional way, garnish each serving with minced fresh parsley and a chunk or two of corn on the cob. Enjoy with crusty bread.

Cream of Mushroom Soup

Yield: 4 to 6 servings

This is one of my husband's old favorites.

Per serving: Calories 160, Protein 8 g, Soy Protein 6 g, Fat 8 g, Carbohydrates 11 g

2 tablespoons nondairy margarine

2 medium onions, minced

2 cloves garlic, minced

1½ cups thinly sliced crimini (brown button) mushrooms

Salt, to taste

4 cups vegetarian broth

1 bay leaf

1 teaspoon each dried thyme and tarragon

1 pound medium-firm tofu

1½ cups water

2 tablespoons potato starch

Freshly ground pepper, to taste

Pinch of freshly grated nutmeg

¼ cup chopped fresh parsley

Melt the margarine in a medium pot over medium-high heat. Add the onions and garlic, and sauté for a couple of minutes. Add the mushrooms and sauté about 5 minutes, salting to taste, until the juices have evaporated. Add broth, bay leaf, thyme, and tarragon, and simmer for 10 minutes.

Meanwhile, in a blender or food processor, purée the tofu, water, and potato starch until very smooth. Add to the mushroom mixture, reduce the heat to low, and stir until slightly thickened. Add salt, pepper, and nutmeg to taste. Serve each bowl with a sprinkling of parsley on top.

Chapter 10

Lunch, supper, and side dishes

These are some of our favorite soy dishes—quick, versatile, easy, and delicious enough to serve almost any time of day. Many of these have proven to be hits with children and teens too. Several of these recipes would make delicious soy-rich, vegetarian "fast food" alternatives in restaurants or cafes: the Best Ever Tofu Burgers, Arabic Pizzas, Teriyaki Tofu Burgers, Soyfelafel, Ramen Noodles Plus, and Japanese Tofu Patties, for instance.

Teriyaki Tofu Burgers

Yield: about 8 burgers

Serve these like cutlets or as burgers on sesame buns. You also can slice them up and eat in a wheat tortilla, or add them to a stir-fry. This marinade also can be used on reconstituted textured soy protein chunks and commercial vegetarian chicken-style products.

Per burger: Calories 118, Protein 8 g, Soy Protein 8 g, Fat 4 g, Carbohydrates 11 g

1½ pounds firm regular tofu

Teriyaki Marinade:

½ cup soy sauce

½ cup water

¼ cup dry sherry, white wine, or apple, pineapple, or white grape juice

⅓ cup maple syrup or unbleached sugar

1 teaspoon grated fresh ginger, or ¼ teaspoon powdered ginger

1 clove garlic, crushed

Cut the tofu into ¼-inch-thick slices.

In a small saucepan, mix together the marinade ingredients. Simmer over high heat for a few minutes until cooked through. Lay the tofu slices in a shallow container, and pour the sauce over them. Cover and refrigerate for up to a week. Grill or broil the slices, or pan-fry in a nonstick skillet over medium-high heat until browned on both sides.

Best-Ever *Tofu Burgers*

Yield: 6 large burgers

I've tried many tofu burgers, and while many taste fine, I miss the chewy texture and juiciness associated with a truly good burger. In this burger (from my first book The Almost No-Fat Cookbook*), frozen tofu provides the chewiness, and the dark marinade lends a meaty flavor and moist juices. If you have access to Marmite, the yeast extract paste popular in England and Canada as a spread for toast, by all means try it in this recipe. Its dark, rich flavor adds the perfect touch.*

Per burger: Calories 129, Protein 11 g, Soy Protein 11 g, Fat 7 g, Carbohydrates 6 g

2 pounds medium-firm or firm tofu,
  frozen at least 48 hours

Marinade:

1½ cups water

2 tablespoons dark soy sauce

2 tablespoons ketchup

2 teaspoons Marmite, yeast extract, or
  dark miso

¼ teaspoon garlic granules

¼ teaspoon dried oregano

¼ teaspoon dried basil

¼ teaspoon onion powder

2 teaspoons Kitchen Bouquet or other
  gravy browner (optional)

Thaw the tofu (see page 55). Cut each pound block into 3 thick slices. Cover a cookie sheet with a couple of clean, folded tea towels, and place the slices on top. Cover the slices with more tea towels and another cookie sheet. Place a heavy weight, such as a dictionary or brick, on top of the cookie sheet, and leave for about 15 to 20 minutes.

In a small bowl, mix all the marinade ingredients. Place the tofu slices in a single layer in a shallow pan, and pour the marinade over the slices. Cover and let marinate in the refrigerator for several hours or days.

Just before serving, sauté the slices in a nonstick skillet or lightly oiled, heavy-bottom skillet over medium-high heat until browned on both sides. Serve on buns with all the trimmings.

Japanese Tofu Patties

Yield: 8 to 12 patties

This simple tofu dish, called "Ganmodoki," is made every day in tofu shops in Japan, using the remaining tofu made the day before. These patties are usually deep-fried, but they can be successfully sautéed or oven-baked. They are delicious cold or hot and will keep one week in the refrigerator. They make great snacks and hiking food too.

Per patty: Calories 37, Protein 3 g, Soy Protein 2 g, Fat 2 g, Carbohydrates 2 g

1¼ to 1½ cups crumbled firm tofu

2 tablespoons grated carrot

⅛ cup grated fresh ginger

2 tablespoons minced onion, green onion, or leek

⅛ cup frozen baby peas, thawed

2 tablespoons lightly toasted sesame seeds

¾ teaspoon salt

⅛ cup chopped mushrooms, preferably shiitake or dried, soaked Chinese mushrooms (optional)

Vegetable oil, for frying

Bright Idea: You can use large patties as you would regular burgers, or small patties as appetizers. Eat them plain or with soy sauce, chutney, ketchup, or salsa. Cold tofu patties can also be sliced and added to Japanese-style soups and stews (oden). Or braise whole cold patties for 4 to 5 minutes in a mixture of 4 cups water, ¼ cup Japanese soy sauce, ¼ cup dry sherry or mirin (Japanese rice wine), and 1 tablespoon unbleached sugar.

Combine all the ingredients and knead together by hand or in a food processor until the mixture holds together. Form into 8 to 12 patties (or more tiny ones for appetizers) with smooth edges.

To sauté, heat about ½ inch of vegetable oil in a frying pan over medium-high heat. Add the patties and fry until golden and crispy on the bottom. Turn over and fry until the other side is golden and crispy. Drain on paper towels.

To oven-bake, preheat the oven to 500°F. Place the patties on oiled dark cookie sheets (which help foods brown better), and brush or spray with a little vegetable oil. Bake about 6 minutes per side, or until golden and crispy on both sides and slightly puffed up.

Ecuadorean Potato Cakes
with Peanut Sauce

Yield: 6 to 8 servings

Here is another inventive South American potato dish (Llapingachos Con Salsa De Mano). Tofu replaces fresh cheese, with excellent results. This recipe of mine first appeared in the March 1994 Vegetarian Times.

Per serving: Calories 281, Protein 10 g, Soy Protein 5 g, Fat 10 g, Carbohydrates 37 g

Peanut Sauce:

1 tablespoon extra-virgin olive oil

2 cloves garlic, minced

1 medium onion, minced

Pinch of paprika

2 medium tomatoes, chopped, or 1 cup canned diced tomatoes (reserve the juice)

¼ cup peanut butter mixed with ½ cup hot water

½ cup hot tomato juice (or juice from canned tomatoes) or water

½ teaspoon salt

¼ teaspoon cayenne

Freshly ground black pepper, to taste

Potato Cakes:

2 pounds Yukon Gold potatoes, peeled and cut into chunks

2 teaspoons extra-virgin olive oil

2 onions, minced

1 clove garlic, minced

Pinch of paprika

2 cups crumbled firm tofu

¾ teaspoon salt

Freshly ground black pepper, to taste

Garnish:

Lettuce leaves

Tomato wedges

Avocado slices drizzled with fresh lemon juice

To make the peanut sauce, heat the olive oil in a medium saucepan over medium-high heat. Sauté the 2 cloves garlic, 1 medium onion, paprika, and tomatoes. When the onions are soft, add the diluted peanut butter, tomato juice or water, salt, cayenne, and black pepper. Stir and simmer until thickened and hot. Keep warm.

To make the potato cakes, boil the potatoes in salted water until tender. Drain and mash. Set aside.

Heat the olive oil in a medium saucepan over medium-high heat. Sauté the onion, garlic, and paprika until the onions are very soft, adding a little water if necessary to keep from sticking. Add the onions and tofu to the mashed potatoes. Mix well and form into 12 to 16 patties, about ½-inch thick. Cook the patties over medium heat in a lightly oiled non-stick skillet until browned on both sides. Top each serving with hot peanut sauce, and garnish with lettuce, tomatoes, and avocado slices.

Soyfelafel

The tofu keeps these soft and moist inside even though they are baked. The quick baking at high heat makes them crispy on the outside.

Per 2 balls: Calories 93, Protein 5 g, Soy Protein 2 g, Fat 2 g, Carbohydrates 14 g

1 medium onion

1 cup chopped fresh parsley,   or
  ½ cup chopped fresh parsley plus
  ½ cup chopped fresh cilantro or
  mint

5 cloves garlic

1 cup cooked or canned drained
  chick-peas

½ pound medium-firm tofu

1½ cups loosely packed fresh
  bread crumbs

1 tablespoon lemon juice

2 teaspoons ground cumin

1½ teaspoons ground coriander

1 teaspoon salt

¼ teaspoon cayenne

Freshly ground black pepper, to
  taste

Preheat the oven to 500°F. In a food processor, finely mince the onion, parsley, and garlic. Add the remaining ingredients and process briefly. Drop heaping tablespoonfuls onto 2 cookie sheets oiled with olive oil. Flatten each mound a little with an oiled spoon, keeping the edges of the patties as smooth and even as possible. Bake in the hot oven for 5 to 7 minutes or until golden brown and crispy on the bottom. Turn the patties over and bake another 5 to 7 minutes or until the both sides are crispy and golden brown.

Serve in fresh whole-wheat pita breads with either dark greens, such as arugula and Romaine lettuce, or sliced cucumber, tomato, and onion, and Tofu Herb Sauce (see page 98) along with some hot sauce.

If you'd like the patties to have a little more of a fried flavor, you can let them cool and then sauté them briefly in a nonstick skillet with about ½ to 1 tablespoon olive oil for each 7 or 8 balls.

Arabic Pizzas

Traditionally, these Arabic, Lebanese, or Armenian meat pies consist of pita bread dough baked with a topping of minced meat, tomatoes, and herbs. Here, the topping is made with vegetarian burger instead and is baked on top of purchased soft pita bread for ease and convenience—and they are delicious! These make a great light lunch too.

Per serving: Calories 328, Protein 16 g, Soy Protein 7 g, Fat 6 g,
Carbohydrates 55 g

6 fresh soft pita breads

Filling:

1 small onion, minced

½ cup chopped canned tomatoes, drained

About 1½ cups commercial vegetarian hamburger crumbles or reconstituted beef-style textured soy protein

¼ cup chopped minced parsley

1 teaspoon lemon juice

½ teaspoon ground cumin

¼ teaspoon salt

Liquid red pepper sauce and black pepper, to taste

Tofu Sour Cream or Yogurt (page 97), or Soy Yogurt (page 86), or a commercial version, for garnish

Preheat the oven to 400°F.

To make the filling, sauté or steam-fry (see page 67) the onion with a little oil or tomato juice from the canned tomatoes until softened. Mix in the remaining filling ingredients, and sauté briefly to heat and mix well. Spread the filling evenly over the 6 pita breads, and place them on ungreased cookie sheets. Bake for 10 minutes or until the bottoms are slightly crispy. Serve hot or at room temperature with Tofu Sour Cream or Yogurt, Soy Yogurt, or a commercial soy yogurt to spread on top. The pizzas can also be topped with grilled eggplant for a quick meal.

Vegetarian Quiche Lorraine

Yield: one 9-inch quiche or four 4-inch individual quiches

This is really delicious, as smooth and rich-tasting as the real thing! Custard powder is a cornstarched-based thickener popular in Canada that has the color of custard. If unavailable in your area, use the cornstarch and saffron alternative listed here.

Per small quiche: Calories 131, Protein 10 g, Soy Protein 10 g, Fat 6 g, Carbohydrates 8 g

One 9-inch pie shell, or four 4-inch pie shells

4 slices vegetarian ham or Canadian bacon, or about 8 slices vegetarian bacon

¼ cup soy Parmesan

1¾ cups soymilk

½ cup medium-firm tofu

1 chicken-style vegetarian bouillon cube, crumbled, or enough broth powder for 1 cup liquid

1½ tablespoons cornstarch or wheat starch, plus a pinch of Spanish saffron, or 1 tablespoon custard powder plus ½ tablespoon cornstarch

½ teaspoon agar powder, or 1 tablespoon agar flakes

½ teaspoon salt

Pinch each of pepper and nutmeg

For a wheat- and corn-free version, omit the custard powder and cornstarch and use 2¼ tablespoons white rice flour and a pinch of Spanish saffron (for a yellower color). Use your favorite wheat-free crust recipe.

For more body, with or without the veggie ham or bacon, add lightly steamed, well-drained vegetables, such as asparagus or broccoli. You can also use ½ cup slivered smoked tofu instead of the ham. Chopped fresh herbs can also be added.

Preheat the oven to 425°F for a 9-inch quiche or 400°F for individual quiches.

Prick the crust all over, and bake for 5 minutes. Remove from the oven.

Brown the ham or bacon in a nonstick pan. Slice it thinly and scatter over the bottom of the pastry.

Process the remaining ingredients in a blender until smooth, and pour into the crust. Bake for 10 minutes, then cover the edges of the pastry with strips of foil, and bake 20 minutes more. (Bake individual quiches at 400°F for 25 minutes.)

The quiche needs to be cooled at least to room temperature to be firm. It will keep well in the refrigerator for a few days.

30-Minute *Vegetarian Chili*

Yield: 6 generous servings

Despite the speed of preparation, this is very authentic-tasting chili.

Per serving: Calories 345, Protein 22 g, Soy Protein 10 g, Fat 3 g,
Carbohydrates 57 g

1 tablespoon extra-virgin olive oil

6 cloves garlic, chopped or crushed

3 tablespoons chili powder (preferably a dark one, such as ancho)

1 tablespoon dried oregano

½ tablespoon ground cumin

½ teaspoon dried red chili flakes

One 28-ounce can diced tomatoes and juice

4½ cups cooked or canned pinto beans (about three 15-ounce cans, drained)

3 cups hot water or bean broth from home-cooked beans (don't use the more salty canned bean liquid)

1½ cups dry textured soy protein granules

¼ cup soy sauce

1 tablespoon liquid hot pepper sauce

1 tablespoon onion powder

1 tablespoon unsweetened cocoa powder

1 teaspoon sugar

1 green bell pepper, seeded and chopped (optional)

1 cup corn kernels (optional)

1 cup or more diced summer squash (optional)

½ teaspoon salt, or to taste

2 tablespoons cornmeal or masa harina

In a large pot, sauté the garlic in the olive oil over medium heat until it just begins to turn color. Add the chili powder, oregano, cumin, and chili flakes, and cook for a couple of minutes more. Add all of the remaining ingredients, except the salt and cornmeal.

Simmer for about 20 minutes. During the last 5 minutes, sprinkle the cornmeal or masa harina over the top, and stir it in.

Add salt to taste.

Serve with rice, bread, polenta, tortillas, or cornbread. This freezes well.

You can substitute about 2 cups squeezed, crumbled, frozen firm tofu for the textured soy protein. In this case, reduce the water or bean liquid to 1½ cups instead of 3 cups.

Mac and Cheese

Yield: 4 to 6 servings

This is really good! One caution: Although you may think it looks like too much sauce, the pasta really soaks it up. You can find the calcium carbonate used in this recipe at your local pharmacy.

Per serving: Calories 271, Protein 113 g, Soy Protein 2 g, Fat 1 g, Carbohydrates 48 g

12 ounces penne, rigatoni, or medium shell pasta

Sauce:

2 cups water

⅔ cup nutritional yeast flakes

⅔ cup extra-firm silken tofu or medium-firm regular tofu

⅓ cup unbleached flour

¼ cup cornstarch

1 chicken-style vegetarian bouillon cube, crumbled, or enough broth powder to flavor 1 cup liquid

3 tablespoons calcium carbonate powder (optional)

2 tablespoons light miso

2 teaspoons lemon juice

½ to ¾ teaspoon salt

1 teaspoon vegetarian Worcestershire sauce, or ½ teaspoon each garlic granules, Hungarian paprika, dry mustard, and Tabasco sauce

¼ teaspoon white pepper

2 cups water

Pinch of freshly ground nutmeg

1 to 2 tablespoons nondairy margarine (optional)

1 cup fresh bread crumbs

Paprika

Soy Parmesan, for garnish

Cook the pasta until al dente. Drain and set aside.

Preheat the oven to 350°F. Combine all of the sauce ingredients except the last 2 cups water, the nutmeg, and margarine, if using, and the bread crumbs and paprika. Blend until very smooth. Pour into a large pot or microwave-proof bowl, and whisk in the remaining 2 cups water.

Place the pot over medium heat, and stir until the mixture thickens. Turn the heat down and cook for several minutes, stirring frequently.

To microwave, cook 4 minutes, and whisk. Microwave 4 minutes more, whisk, and microwave 3 minutes more.

Whisk in the nutmeg and margarine, if using. Add the cooked, drained pasta, and mix well. Spread the mixture in an oiled casserole, and top with bread crumbs and paprika. You can also sprinkle on some soy Parmesan. Bake for about 20 minutes, or until bubbly.

Vegan Corn Custard

Yield: 4 servings

This is a very comforting old-fashioned dish. If you use frozen corn, try to use the peaches-and-cream variety.

Per serving: Calories 157, Protein 9 g, Soy Protein 6 g, Fat 4 g, Carbohydrates 21 g

¾ **pound medium-firm tofu**

3 **tablespoons flour**

1 **tablespoon nutritional yeast flakes**

½ **teaspoon each salt and tumeric**

¼ **teaspoon baking powder**

1 **tablespoon light miso (optional)**

⅛ **teaspoon cayenne (optional)**

2 **cups corn kernels (thawed, if frozen)**

Preheat the oven to 350°F.

Blend together all the ingredients, except the corn kernels, until very smooth. Mix in a bowl with the corn kernels. Spread in an oiled 9-inch pie pan, and bake for 30 to 40 minutes, or until set. Serve warm.

Quesadillas

Quesadillas are tortillas grilled or sautéed with a filling inside, like a turnover. They are not heavily filled—in fact, they should be quite thin—so they make a great light meal or snack.

Preheat the oven to 500°F. For each quesadilla, spread one half of a corn or wheat tortilla with Melty Soy Pizza Cheese (page 103), some crumbled Ricotta Salata (page 106), or grated soy cheese. If you like, add some cooked, mashed beans or commercial vegetarian refried beans. You also can add:

small amounts of canned green or
   jalapeño chilis
chopped fresh tomatoes
chopped oil-packed sun-dried tomatoes
chopped roasted red pepper
chopped cilantro
sliced papaya, mango, pineapple, or
   avocado

green onions
commercial sliced, marinated or
   smoked tofu or cooked tempeh
grilled mushrooms or other vegetables
crumbled soy-based vegetarian sausage
   or chorizo
hamburger substitute
sautéed greens, sautéed mushrooms,
   or corn

Fold over the other half of the tortilla. Either bake on cookie sheets for 5 to 7 minutes until crispy, grill over hot coals until crispy on both sides, or pan-fry in a hot, dry nonstick or cast-iron skillet until crispy on both sides. If you aren't worried about fat, you can use a little oil. Serve with Tofu Sour Cream (page 97) and salsa.

Spanikopita Rolls

Yield: about 48 rolls

The filling for these "little Greek spinach-filo pies" is a bit unusual, containing such un-Greek ingredients as tofu, nutritional yeast, and miso. But these ingredients give the filling a rich, feta-like taste, which is what you expect from spanikopita. I took these to a potluck once, and they were gobbled up before the hostess even got to taste one—no one even suspected that they were nondairy! If you use frozen chopped spinach, the filling takes only minutes to make and can be made a day or two ahead of time, although you should fill and bake the rolls shortly before serving.

Per 3 rolls: Calories 150, Protein 6 g, Soy Protein 3 g, Fat 7 g, Carbohydrates 17 g

12 full sheets of filo pastry, thawed and kept covered

¼ to ½ cup olive oil or melted nondairy margarine

Filling:

¼ cup light miso

1 teaspoon salt

2 tablespoons nutritional yeast flakes

1 bunch green onions, chopped and steam-fried (see page 67) until soft

2 tablespoons dry dill, or ½ cup chopped fresh dill

Three 10-ounce packages frozen chopped spinach, thawed and squeezed dry, or 3 pounds fresh spinach, cleaned, steamed, squeezed dry, and chopped

1½ pounds medium-firm tofu, drained and crumbled

This filling can be used in a savory pie, by the way, with a bottom or double crust, or as a filling for calzone (Italian stuffed breads using pizza dough). You can also make a 9 x 13-inch rectangular spanikopita using ½ pound of filo pastry in a baking dish and baking at 350°F for 40 minutes.

Prepare the filling by mixing the tofu, miso, salt, and yeast together very well in a large bowl. Use your hands, a potato masher, or a fork. Add the dill, green onions, and spinach, and mix well.

To fill the rolls, stack 3 sheets of filo together, and cut the stack into four 6 x 5-inch rectangles with a pair of kitchen scissors or a sharp knife. Repeat with the remaining filo. You should have 48 rectangles. Keep the filo well-covered with plastic wrap while you work. Preheat the oven to 400°F.

For each spanikopita, lightly brush a filo rectangle with olive oil or melted margarine. Place about 3 tablespoons of filling in one corner of the rectangle. Roll the filled corner toward the center, then fold in the left and right corners, like an envelope, then roll up the remaining corner. Cover the filled spanikopita with plastic wrap while you finish.

Place the filled rolls, seam-side-down, on nonstick or lightly oiled cookie sheets. Brush or spray the tops lightly with olive oil or melted margarine. Bake for 20 minutes, or until golden brown. Serve hot.

Ramen Noodles Plus

Yield: 2 to 3 servings

This recipe makes a real meal out of instant ramen noodles.

Per serving: Calories 381, Protein 13 g, Soy Protein 8 g, Fat 5 g, Carbohydrates 24 g

2 packages instant vegetarian ramen noodles, including the powdered soup base packet

4 cups water

½ pound broccoli or other vegetable, sliced and cooked until crisp-tender

3 to 4 green onions, sliced

5 triangles Oven-Fried Tofu (page 110), sliced into strips

½ cup frozen baby peas or whole green beans

Toasted sesame oil, for garnish

Follow the directions on the package for making the soup. Add all the remaining ingredients, sprinkling the toasted sesame oil on each serving as a garnish.

Chapter 11

Dinner entrees

This chapter contains many of our favorite family dishes. It is a truly international collection and shows clearly how adaptable soyfoods are to the cuisines of the world. You can sample curries and stir-fries; stews from Italy, France, and Ireland; Mexican-American specialties; kebabs from Japan and India; sophisticated Italian pasta dishes; an Argentinean shepherd's pie; and comfort foods from North America—all featuring soyfoods as the main protein source.

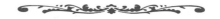

Soy and Seitan Turkey

Yield: 4 seitan turkey breast halves or 1 large roasted turkey breast (enough for 8 to 12 servings)

This recipe makes outstanding sandwiches. Try it with vegetarian ham or Canadian bacon for club sandwiches. The instant gluten powder is also called vital wheat gluten and is available at some natural food stores and through the sources on page 184.

Per serving: Calories 205, Protein 32 g, Soy Protein 5 g, Fat 3 g, Carbohydrates 12 g

Broth:

8 cups water

1 cup chopped onion, or ¼ cup dried onion flakes

⅓ cup nutritional yeast flakes

3 tablespoons light soy sauce

2½ teaspoons salt

½ teaspoon dried thyme

½ teaspoon dried rosemary

½ teaspoon dried sage

Tofu Mix:

¾ pound firm tofu

1½ cups water

3 tablespoons light soy sauce

Dry Mix:

2 cups instant gluten powder (vital wheat gluten)

½ cup full-fat soy flour

½ cup nutritional yeast flakes

2 teaspoons onion powder

¾ teaspoon garlic granules

¼ teaspoon white pepper

Mix the broth ingredients in a large pot, and bring to a boil.

In a food processor, blend all the tofu mix ingredients until smooth. Add all the dry mix ingredients to the tofu mix, and process briefly until the mixture forms a ball on the blade. Remove and, with wet hands, form into four 1-inch-thick ovals. With a slotted spoon, lower the ovals gently into the boiling broth, reduce the heat, cover, and simmer gently for 1 hour, turning and piercing the pieces with a fork every now and then. Cool in the cooking broth. Tightly cover and store in the cooking broth in the refrigerator or freezer.

Slice the seitan turkey very thinly for sandwiches, into ¼-inch-thick cutlets for scaloppine, into chunks for stews and pot pies, slivers for stir-fries, or oblong chunks for mock fried chicken or other chicken dishes, browning the chunks first in a little oil.

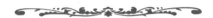

Roasted Turkey Breast

Before cooking the soy and seitan turkey in broth, shape the mixture into one large oval shape no more than 2 inches thick. Cook as directed. Preheat the oven to 350°F. Place the cooked seitan turkey breast in a shallow, oiled baking dish. Add about ½ cup of the cooking broth to the bottom of the pan. Baste with a mixture of 3 tablespoons olive oil, 1 tablespoon toasted sesame oil, and 1 clove crushed garlic.

Bake for about 45 to 60 minutes, basting with the oil mixture until golden brown on the outside. Add a little more cooking broth if the pan becomes dry. (You can bake your favorite vegetarian stuffing in a casserole or loaf or tube pan at the same time.)

Serve with mashed potatoes, cranberry sauce, and Brown Yeast Gravy (page 104) or your favorite vegetarian gravy, perhaps with mushrooms added, and any of your other traditional holiday dishes.

If you want a golden skin on the turkey, you can use yuba (Chinese bean curd skin sheets—see page 57). Soak the largest of the fragile sheets for at least 5 minutes in warm water until they are pliable. Wrap the cooked turkey breast with 2 or 3 layers of yuba, tucking it under the turkey. Baste every 15 minutes with the basting mixture. If it browns too quickly, cover loosely with foil. Let stand 10 to 15 minutes before serving.

Grilled Yakitori Skewers

Yield: 8 servings

Traditionally, yakitori are little skewers of chicken and chicken liver with a sticky Japanese soy glaze. Here we skewer chunks of extra-firm tofu and mushrooms. You also could substitute tempeh or reconstituted textured soy protein chunks for the tofu. This makes great fare for a barbecue or picnic.

You can purchase bamboo skewers in most large supermarkets or hardware stores, or in Asian grocery stores or cookware shops. Soak the skewers in water for 15 minutes before using them, to prevent burning.

Per serving: Calories 141, Protein 9 g, Soy Protein 8 g, Fat 4 g, Carbohydrates 16 g

¾ cup soy sauce

¾ cup dry sherry or mirin (Japanese rice wine)

4½ tablespoons unbleached sugar

1½ pounds extra-firm tofu, cut into 72 cubes

16 bamboo skewers

32 small fresh button mushrooms, preferably criminis

About 16 green onions, trimmed to include only 3 inches of the green part and cut into 1½-inch lengths

3 tablespoons cornstarch mixed with ⅓ cup cold water

Mix together the soy sauce, sugar, and sherry or mirin in a small saucepan over high heat until the sugar dissolves. Place the tofu cubes in a shallow dish, and pour the soy sauce mixture over them. Marinate in the refrigerator for several hours or days, stirring or shaking once in a while.

When ready to cook, thread the marinated tofu cubes on the soaked skewers, alternating with the mushrooms and green onion pieces.

Pour the remaining marinade into a small saucepan, and add the dissolved cornstarch and water. Stir over high heat until the sauce thickens and boils.

Spur-of-the-Moment Kebabs

Follow the recipe for Grilled Yakitori Skewers, but substitute any barbecue sauce or glaze that you like. You can use your favorite homemade or commercial one; even a flavorful fat-free vinaigrette works.

Instead of, or in addition to, the mushrooms and green onions, you can use small partially cooked red potatoes, bell pepper pieces, small quartered onions, eggplant, zucchini, or pineapple chunks, and so forth.

Brush the skewers with the sauce, and grill or broil about 3 to 4 inches from the heat source until glazed and slightly charred on all sides (about 7 minutes). Baste with the glaze when you turn the skewers.

Serve the skewers immediately with steamed rice.

Tandoori Kebabs Yield: 4 servings

These scrumptious kebabs can be easily made in your oven broiler at any time of the year, or on a hibachi, indoor grill, or barbecue.

Per serving: Calories 157, Protein 11 g, Soy Protein 8 g, Fat 5 g, Carbohydrates 15 g

Tandoori Marinade:

1 cup Tofu Yogurt (page 97)

2 medium onions, diced

4 teaspoons ground ginger

2 teaspoons turmeric

1 teaspoon curry powder

1 teaspoon chili powder

½ teaspoon each ground
coriander, cumin, garlic granules,
nutmeg and paprika

¾ pound extra-firm tofu, or
14 ounces pressed tofu, cut into
48 equal cubes and marinated at
least 12 hours in Breast of Tofu
Marinade (page 144)

32 small mushroom caps

8 bamboo skewers, soaked in cold
water at least 15 minutes

In a shallow container or dish, mix together the tandoori marinade ingredients. Add the tofu cubes, mixing well and making sure the tofu cubes are covered. Cover and marinate for several hours or several days, in the refrigerator.

Thread the tofu cubes and mushroom caps alternately on the skewers. Broil, grill, or barbecue the skewers, basting with the marinade occasionally, until slightly charred on two sides. Serve hot in chapatis, whole-wheat pita breads, or flour tortillas, with Tofu Sour Cream or Yogurt (page 97), chutney, and perhaps sliced raw vegetables on the side.

Saag Panir with Tofu

This is a well-loved Indian dish that usually is made with fresh Indian cheese called panir. Tofu works beautifully in this dish, and a little olive oil stands in for ghee (clarified butter). The garam masala called for here is a blend of common spices used in Indian cooking. It can be purchased at specialty or natural food stores, and the spices used can vary from brand to brand. Serve saag panir with steamed basmati rice and/or whole-wheat chapatis, or even tortillas.

Per serving: Calories 151, Protein 10 g, Soy Protein 7 g, Fat 7 g, Carbohydrates 11 g

1 pound firm tofu, cut in ½-inch cubes

¼ cup medium-firm regular tofu or firm or extra-firm silken tofu

½ cup water

2 teaspoons lemon juice

1 tablespoon extra-virgin olive oil

1½ cups minced onion

2 tablespoons grated fresh ginger

2 tablespoons minced pickled jalapeños

2 teaspoons garam masala or curry powder

1 teaspoon salt

½ teaspoon turmeric

Two 10-ounce packages frozen chopped spinach, thawed and drained

Cook the tofu cubes in a nonstick skillet without any oil over medium heat until golden on all sides. Remove from the pan and set aside.

Bright Idea: If you are short of time and don't mind the extra oil, substitute 2 cups of diced commercial Japanese fried tofu cubes or triangles (atsuage) for the firm tofu.

Meanwhile, process the ¼ cup tofu with the water and lemon juice in a blender until smooth; set aside.

Add the olive oil to the pan. When the oil is hot, add the onion. Sauté until the onions are tender, adding a little water if necessary to keep them from sticking. Add the ginger and jalapeños, and cook for 2 minutes. Add the garam masala or curry powder, salt, and turmeric, and sauté for a minute.

Add the cooked tofu cubes, spinach, and the blended tofu mixture to the onion mixture. Simmer gently for about 4 minutes. Add salt to taste and serve immediately.

Vegan Tuna-Noodle Casserole

Yield: 4 servings

This needs little introduction. Most of us who grew up in North America in the '50s, '60s, and '70s know this casserole well! Despite the jokes about it, kids love it and adults find it comforting and familiar. I think this version is better than the original.

Per serving: Calories 348, Protein 17 g, Soy Protein 11 g, Fat 15 g, Carbohydrates 35 g

6 ounces bow-tie pasta

1 tablespoon extra-virgin olive oil

1 medium onion, chopped

2 cloves garlic, chopped

½ pound oyster or white button mushrooms, sliced

½ cup chopped celery

2 cups (one recipe) thin Nondairy Bechamel (pages 96-97)

1 cup frozen baby peas, thawed under hot water and drained

1 cup medium-firm tofu, cut into small dice and drained well

¼ cup chopped roasted red peppers (homemade or commercial)

Pinch each of dill, celery seed, and pepper

1 tablespoon dulse flakes

½ teaspoon kelp powder (optional)

Salt and freshly ground black pepper, to taste

2 tablespoons dry sherry (optional)

1 cup fresh bread crumbs

¼ cup soy Parmesan

Paprika, for garnish

Preheat the oven to 375°F.

Boil the pasta until al dente, then drain.

Heat the olive oil in a medium pan over medium heat. Add the onion, garlic, mushrooms, and celery, and sauté until softened. Remove from the heat and add the cooked pasta and remaining ingredients, except the bread crumbs, soy Parmesan, and paprika. Mix well and add salt and pepper to taste. Spoon into a shallow, oiled 2-quart casserole, and sprinkle the bread crumbs, soy Parmesan, and a little paprika over the top. Bake for 30 to 35 minutes.

Savory Tofu Dinner Loaf

Yield: 6 servings

If you're craving good old American meat loaf, you are in for a treat. This simple recipe is amazingly good, hot or cold, and makes delicious sandwiches. The little bit of instant gluten powder called for in the recipe gives it a wonderfully chewy texture. Often called vital wheat gluten, you can find this in many natural food stores or through some of the sources on page 184. You can also try different seasonings in this recipe, if you like. You can double the recipe to make 2 loaves or bake the mixture in 12 muffin cups for about 20 minutes.

Per serving: Calories 155, Protein 15 g, Soy Protein 9 g, Fat 5 g, Carbohydrates 11 g

1 cup fresh whole-wheat bread crumbs

⅓ cup water or wine

2 cups minced onions (2 large onions)

2 cloves garlic, minced

1½ pounds frozen, medium-firm tofu, thawed, squeezed dry, and crumbled (page 55)

¼ cup soy sauce

½ tablespoon tomato paste, or 1 tablespoon ketchup

1 teaspoon gravy browner, such as Kitchen Bouquet

½ teaspoon each dried basil, sage, and oregano

¼ teaspoon each dried thyme and savory

Freshly ground black pepper, to taste

¼ cup instant gluten powder (vital wheat gluten)

In a large bowl, mix together the bread crumbs and water or wine. Set aside.

In a large, lightly oiled or nonstick skillet, cook the onions and garlic slowly over medium heat, adding a little water as necessary to keep from sticking, until the onions are very soft, but before they are beginning to brown. This is very important to the taste and texture of the dish, so don't undercook them. Or microwave the onions and garlic in a covered dish or casserole on high for 10 minutes.

Preheat the oven to 350°F. Add the onions to the bread crumbs along with the tofu, soy sauce, tomato paste or ketchup, herbs, gravy browner, and pepper to taste. Mix well and allow the mixture to cool thoroughly. If you don't cool the mixture, the gluten powder will turn stringy when you add it; you can speed up the cooling by spreading the mixture on a cookie sheet and placing it in the freezer for a few minutes.

Add the gluten powder and mix well. Pat the mixture into a lightly greased or nonstick 9-inch-round cake or pie pan. If you like, spread the top with a thin layer of ketchup, tomato sauce, or barbecue sauce. Bake 30 minutes, then let the loaf sit for 10 to 15 minutes before cutting into wedges. It firms up more when cold.

Old-Fashioned Brown Stew

Yield: 6 to 8 servings

Serve this hearty vegetarian stew with boiled potatoes, mashed potatoes, crusty bread, or even rice or eggless broad noodles. Leftovers can be made into pot pie or Cornish-style savory turnovers made with Low-Fat Pastry Crust (pages 160-61) or your favorite biscuit dough.

Per serving: Calories 174, Protein 14 g, Soy Protein 10 g, Fat 0 g, Carbohydrates 28 g

1½ cups dry textured soy protein chunks (see page 54)

2 medium onions, sliced

1 clove garlic, minced

⅓ cup unbleached flour

5 cups water

4 to 5 cups peeled, cubed vegetables (such as mushrooms, celery, eggplant, red or green bell pepper, carrot, parsnip, rutabaga, and turnip)

½ cup dry red lentils

¼ cup soy sauce

¼ cup tomato paste

1 teaspoon unbleached sugar

3 to 4 vegetarian bouillon cubes, or enough broth powder to flavor 3 to 4 cups liquid

1 bay leaf

2 teaspoons Marmite, yeast extract, or dark miso

¼ teaspoon each dried thyme, rosemary, and marjoram

Freshly ground black pepper, to taste

1 cup frozen baby peas

Gravy browner, such as Kitchen Bouquet

½ cup chopped fresh parsley (optional)

Reconstitute the textured soy chunks in 1½ cups boiling water, either soaking or simmering until tender. (See page 54.) Drain well and pat dry.

In a large, heavy lightly oiled stockpot, steam-fry (see page 67) the onion and garlic over medium heat, adding a little water as necessary to keep them from sticking. When the onions begin to soften and brown, add the flour and stir well. Add all the remaining ingredients except the peas, gravy browner, and parsley. Bring to a boil, then reduce the heat and simmer for at least 30 minutes, or until the vegetables are tender. Add the peas and simmer for 10 more minutes. Add the gravy browner and the parsley, if desired, and add salt to taste.

❧ *Irish Stew:* Omit the garlic, tomato paste, and peas. Use 1 cup Guiness Stout in place of 1 cup water. For vegetables, use only celery, mushrooms, carrots, turnips, and parsnips. Serve with Colcannon (mashed potatoes mixed with chopped steamed kale or other greens).

Italian-Style Stew

Serves 4

Vegetarian proteins do not need long cooking to tenderize, but a couple of hours melds the flavors in this delicious pot of stew nicely. Serve it with mashed potatoes, crusty bread, or polenta. Leftovers are something to look forward to!

This stew recipe can be altered to suit your taste. You can use a dry white wine or white vermouth instead of the red wine. You can add a little more Marmite (yeast extract) for a "beefier" flavor. You can substitute sage or oregano for the rosemary. You can eliminate the tomatoes and add another cup of broth, and then perhaps finish the dish with a little soy "cream" (page 99).

For a little extra tang or spice, you can add a few capers, a dash of lemon juice or balsamic vinegar, black kalamata olives, or a sprinkle of hot pepper flakes at the end. Other vegetables, such as baby onions, fennel, strips of bell peppers (any color) or soaked porcini or boletus mushrooms could also be added.

Per serving: Calories 248, Protein 18 g, Soy Protein 15 g, Fat 5 g, Carbohydrates 28 g

2 cups reconstituted textured soy protein chunks (1½ cups dry—see page 54), well-drained and patted dry

Flour or Seasoned Flour (page 144)

1 tablespoon extra-virgin olive oil

1 teaspoon Chinese roasted sesame oil

1 large onion, chopped

16 medium white button or cremini mushrooms, sliced

1 cup chopped celery with tops

½ carrot, peeled and chopped

Couple of sprigs parsley, chopped (preferably flat leafed Italian)

2 cloves garlic, chopped

One 14 ounce can diced tomatoes with juice

4 carrots, peeled and cut into "fingers"

2 cups water

½ cup dry red wine (or nonalcoholic)

1 vegetarian broth cube (enough for 1 cup broth)

2 teaspoons lite soy sauce

1½ teaspoons Marmite, yeast extract, or dark miso

1 teaspoon dried thyme

½ teaspoon dried rosemary

1 bay leaf

Pinch unbleached sugar

Salt and freshly ground pepper

Minced fresh Italian parsley

Dredge the chunks of soy protein in flour. Heat the oils in a heavy pot or Dutch oven over medium-high heat. Brown the chunks in the oil. Remove and set aside. Add the onion to the pot, and steam-fry, adding a little water as necessary, until the onions start to soften. Add mushrooms, celery, ½ carrot, parsley, and garlic. Steam-fry until the vegetables start to soften.

Add the chunks, tomatoes, carrots, water, wine, bouillon cube, soy sauce, Marmite, herbs, and sugar. Simmer for about 2 hours. Taste for salt and pepper, and sprinkle with parsley.

Apple and Potato Stew

Yield: 4 servings

Before I was a vegetarian, I made this stew with pork. It was so good that I made a vegan version which makes a wonderful fall or winter dish.

Per serving: Calories 418, Protein 19 g, Soy Protein 15 g, Fat 6 g, Carbohydrates 69 g

1½ cups dry textured soy protein chunks

About 1 cup Seasoned Flour (page 144)

1 to 2 tablespoons extra-virgin olive oil or nondairy margarine

3 medium onions, sliced

2 cloves garlic, minced

½ teaspoon paprika

¼ teaspoon pepper

Pinch of rubbed sage

4 large potatoes, cut into sixths (or 6 medium ones, cut in quarters)

2 large apples, cored and cut into chunks (peel only if not organic or if the skins are unsightly)

1½ cups vegetarian broth

2 to 4 tablespoons dry sherry or nonalcoholic sweet white wine

2 teaspoons Marmite, yeast extract, or dark miso

1 teaspoon soy sauce

1 teaspoon salt

1 teaspoon sugar

Reconstitute the textured soy chunks in 1½ cups boiling water, either soaking or simmering until tender. (See page 54.) Drain well and pat dry.

Coat the soy protein chunks with seasoned flour. Heat the oil or margarine in a large, heavy stockpot over medium-high heat. Add the soy protein chunks and sliced onions, and sauté until the onions soften. Add the garlic, paprika, and pepper, and sauté, stirring frequently, for a couple of minutes. Add the remaining ingredients.

Bring to a boil, then reduce the heat and simmer about 30 minutes or until the potatoes are tender. Serve hot with crusty bread and a salad.

Spicy Southern-Fried Tofu

Yield: 6 servings

If you prefer to sauté the tofu in hot oil, go right ahead, but the method I use here makes a great crispy, almost fat-free dish.

Per serving: Calories 251, Protein 12 g, Soy Protein 6 g, Fat 7 g, Carbohydrates 34 g

1 pound firm or medium-firm tofu, cut into about 32 cubes and marinated for at least 12 hours in Breast of Tofu marinade (page 144)

Spicy Flour:

2 cups whole-wheat flour

¼ cup nutritional yeast

2 teaspoons baking powder

2 teaspoons garlic granules

2½ teaspoons salt

2 teaspoons dry mustard powder

½ teaspoon each cayenne and black pepper

Dipping Mixture:

1 cup soymilk

¼ cup soy mayonnaise (commercial or Tofu Mayo, page 90)

2 tablespoons Dijon mustard

1 tablespoon lemon juice

1 tablespoon flour

½ tablespoon onion powder

½ teaspoon each salt and dry mustard powder

¼ teaspoon each cayenne and black pepper

Preheat the oven to 400°F.

Lightly oil 2 dark cookie sheets. (The dark color helps brown foods better.)

In a large bowl, mix all of the spicy flour ingredients, and set aside. In another large bowl, mix all of the dipping mixture ingredients. Remove the tofu from the marinade with a slotted spoon, and coat the cubes with the spicy flour. Dip the floured cubes in the dipping mixture, coating all over, then roll them again in the spicy flour to coat. You may find this easiest if you use two forks for dredging the cubes in the flour, and two more forks for immersing them in the dipping mixture.

Place the cubes, not touching, on the cookie sheets. Bake for about 10 minutes, or until golden and crispy on the bottom. Turn them and bake for 7 to 10 minutes more until golden all over.

Serve the cubes hot with gravy and mashed potatoes or steamed rice. They are delicious cold too.

Argentine Shepherd's Pie

Yield: 6 to 8 servings

This is one of my favorite winter dishes, also called "pastel de papa." It works best with a commercial hamburger replacement. I use two packages of Yves Ground Round.

Per serving: Calories 308, Protein 8 g, Soy Protein 5 g, Fat 5 g, Carbohydrates 55 g

Topping:

6 large russet or Yukon Gold potatoes, peeled and cut into chunks

¼ cup soymilk

Salt and white pepper, to taste

Paprika

Soy Parmesan substitute or bread crumbs, for topping (optional)

Filling:

1 tablespoon extra-virgin olive oil

1 large onion, minced

1 green or red bell pepper, seeded and diced small

2 cloves garlic, minced

6 cups commercial vegetarian hamburger crumbles or reconstituted beef-style textured soy granules

One 28-ounce can diced tomatoes, drained

1 cup Brown Gravy (page 104)

2 teaspoons ground cumin

2 teaspoons oregano

Salt and pepper, to taste

½ cup raisins (optional)

½ cup sliced green olives (optional)

Boil the potatoes until tender. Drain them and mash with the soymilk and salt and pepper to taste. Set aside.

Preheat the oven to 375°F.

Heat the oil in a large nonstick skillet over medium-high heat, and sauté the onion, garlic, and bell pepper until the onion has softened. Add the hamburger crumbles and sauté for a few minutes. Add the remaining ingredients, mix, and pour into a large casserole or baking pan. Spread the potato mixture over the casserole, and sprinkle with paprika and soy Parmesan or bread crumbs, if desired.

Bake for 20 to 30 minutes until the casserole is heated through.

Bright Idea: To make this in a hurry, use instant mashed potatoes (6 cups of potato flakes mixed with 4 cups of boiling water), then add the soymilk and salt and pepper. Place the filling in 6 to 8 individual casseroles, cover each with the mashed potatoes, sprinkle with paprika, soy Parmesan, or bread crumbs, if desired, and bake at 400°F for about 10 minutes. Brown a little under the broiler, if you like.

Breast of Tofu

Yield: 32 slices

I always have some extra-firm tofu slices marinating to make Breast of Tofu. The slices will keep refrigerated in the marinade for up to two weeks, ready for a quick and delicious meal. They can be cooked plain in a nonstick skillet or coated with seasoned flour and sautéed to make a crispy skin that is delectable hot or cold. Serve Breast of Tofu plain, in salads and sandwiches, or with any sauce that you would use on chicken. Instead of slices, you can marinate cubes for using in kebabs or Tofu and Vegetable Oven-Broiled Stew (page 156).

Per 2 slices: Calories 45, Protein 3 g, Soy Protein 4 g, Fat 1 g, Carbohydrates 2 g

1½ to 2 pounds extra-firm or pressed tofu

Seasoned Flour (page 144, optional)

Marinade:

1½ cups water

¼ cup soy sauce

3 tablespoons nutritional yeast flakes

2 teaspoons dried sage leaves, crumbled, or 2 tablespoons fresh, chopped sage

½ teaspoon dried rosemary, or ½ tablespoon fresh rosemary

½ teaspoon dried thyme, or ½ tablespoon fresh, chopped thyme

½ teaspoon onion powder

Cut the tofu into ¼-inch-thick slices. In a 5-cup container with a tight lid, mix all of the marinade ingredients. Place the tofu slices in the marinade so that they are fairly tightly packed and covered with liquid. Cover and refrigerate for up to two weeks, shaking daily.

For softer slices, cook the tofu slices over medium heat in a nonstick skillet until golden brown on both sides.

Seasoned Flour

Keep some of this in a tightly covered container in the refrigerator; you'll find many uses for it.

Mix together 2 cups whole-wheat or other whole-grain flour, ¼ cup nutritional yeast flakes, 1 teaspoon salt, 1 teaspoon onion powder, if desired, and freshly ground black pepper to taste.

To make crispy slices, coat the tofu slices with seasoned flour. For each batch of 8 to 10 slices, heat about 1 to 2 tablespoons of olive oil or other vegetable oil in a large, heavy-bottomed skillet (such as cast-iron) over medium heat. When the oil is hot, add the slices and cook until golden brown and crispy on the bottom. Swirl the pan if necessary to distribute the oil evenly while cooking. Turn the slices over and continue to cook the other side over medium heat until golden and crispy. Drain thoroughly on paper towels or paper bags, patting to remove excess oil.

Breast of Tofu with rosemary and white wine

Yield: 4 servings

This is extremely quick and easy to make, and one of my all-time favorites for flavor. It reminds me very much of the chicken with white wine that my mother often made when I was a child growing up in a California winery. She used to place steamed rice into the pan in which the chicken had been cooked and scrape up the delicious drippings to mix with the rice. You could do the same with this dish, or serve it with mashed Yukon Gold potatoes. Note that you will need to have tofu that has been marinating for at least a day in Breast of Tofu marinade.

Per serving: Calories 169, Protein 10 g, Soy Protein 6 g, Fat 7 g, Carbohydrates 11 g

¾ pound firm or extra-firm tofu, sliced in ¼-inch-thick slices and marinated for 24 hours in Breast of Tofu marinade (page 144)

½ cup Seasoned Flour (page 144)

1 tablespoon extra-virgin olive oil

3 cups sliced mushrooms, such as white, cremini, or chanterelle

4 cloves garlic, minced

½ cup white wine, such as Riesling

1 cup chicken-style vegetarian broth

2 sprigs fresh rosemary, stripped off the stalk and chopped

Freshly ground black pepper, to taste

Dredge the tofu slices in the seasoned flour. Heat the olive oil in a large nonstick skillet over medium heat. When the oil is hot, arrange the tofu slices in the pan. Cook until one side is golden, then carefully turn them over and cook until the other side is golden. Remove the tofu from the pan, and set aside.

Add the mushrooms and garlic to the pan, and sprinkle with a little salt. Sauté over high heat until the mushrooms start to wilt, adding a tiny bit of water if they seem to be sticking. Add the tofu, wine, broth, and rosemary. Cook over high heat, stirring gently every now and again until the juices form a sauce. Quickly remove from the heat, and grind the fresh pepper over the dish. Serve immediately.

Cannelloni

Cannelloni (stuffed pasta tubes) are one of the most popular Italian dishes served in North America. The most familiar version is Cannelloni alla Napoletana, stuffed pasta tubes with a tomato sauce and cheese topping.

These cannelloni are stuffed with a vegetarian version of the traditional meat and spinach filling, but you can use any crêpe filling you like. This dish is wonderful for company because it can be made ahead of time, and it never fails to please.

Per serving: Calories 502, Protein 20 g, Soy Protein 8 g, Fat 14 g,
Carbohydrates 83 g

"Meat" and Spinach Filling:

2 tablespoons extra-virgin olive oil

2 cups chopped onion

3 cloves garlic, minced

1 pound fresh spinach, steamed, drained, squeezed dry, and chopped, or one 10-ounce package frozen chopped spinach, thawed and squeezed dry

12 to 16 ounces vegetarian hamburger crumbles

1 tablespoon dried oregano or 3 tablespoons chopped fresh oregano

Freshly ground black pepper, to taste

28 to 30 small uncooked egg-free cannelloni shells

3 cups prepared pasta sauce with a handful of chopped fresh basil

1 recipe thick Nondairy Bechamel Sauce (pages 96-97)

¼ to ½ cup soy Parmesan

To make the filling, heat the olive oil in a large nonstick skillet over medium-high heat. Add the onions and sauté until they begin to soften. Add the garlic and sauté a few minutes longer. Add the spinach and sauté for a few minutes. Add the hamburger crumbles or soy granules and oregano, and cook until the mixture is fairly dry. Add pepper to taste and set aside to cool.

Preheat the oven to 350°F.

Boil the cannelloni shells in salted water according to the package directions. Drain and cool until you can handle them.

> *Bright Idea:* Instead of the hamburger crumbles, you can use 3 cups frozen tofu, thawed, crumbled, squeezed, and mixed with ⅓ cup light soy sauce. Or use 2¼ cups textured soy protein granules reconstituted in 1⅞ cups boiling water and mixed with ⅓ cup light soy sauce.

Fill the shells by holding a tube in one hand, covering the bottom with your fingers. Pack with filling with your other hand.

Spread a thin layer of the pasta sauce in the bottom of a shallow 9 x 13-inch baking pan. Place the stuffed shells in a single layer on top. Cover the shells with the tomato sauce, then drizzle with the bechamel and sprinkle with soy Parmesan. Bake for 30 minutes.

Scaloppine Alla Marsala

Yield: 4 servings

This is one of the more traditional Italian scaloppine dishes. Textured soy protein makes a wonderful substitute for veal. Serve with rice, broad eggless noodles, or orzo (tiny pasta granules).

Per serving: Calories 157, Protein 13 g, Soy Protein 13 g, Fat 5 g, Carbohydrates 13 g

2 to 3 cups reconstituted flavored textured soy protein chunks (page 54), well drained and patted dry (this is important)

¼ cup Seasoned Flour (page 144)

2 tablespoons nondairy margarine or extra-virgin olive oil

½ cup marsala, good-quality sherry, or Madeira

1 bay leaf

1 cup vegetarian broth

Salt and freshly ground pepper, to taste

1 lemon, cut into wedges

Dredge the textured soy protein chunks in the seasoned flour. In a heavy nonstick skillet, heat the margarine or olive oil over medium-high heat. Add the textured soy protein chunks, and sauté until browned.

Add the marsala, bay leaf, and broth. Cover and simmer over medium-low heat for about 5 minutes, adding a little water if necessary to keep the chunks from sticking. You should have a nice sauce, not too thin. If it's taking too long to reduce, uncover the pan and raise the heat a little, but watch carefully that the sauce doesn't cook off completely. Sprinkle with salt and pepper to taste. Serve with lemon wedges to squeeze over the scaloppine.

Bright Idea: Add 1 cup of any kind of sliced mushrooms and/or 1 cup of sliced sweet peppers while browning the scaloppine chunks. You also could add a little garlic and some fresh herbs, such as basil, sage, or rosemary.

Other possible additions include sun-dried tomatoes in oil, sautéed leeks, and sliced artichoke hearts.

Lasagne Al Forno Bolognese

Yield: 8 servings

This is the traditional northern Italian lasagne, and my husband invariably requests it for his birthday dinner. The dish consists of pasta, soy Parmesan, and two other recipes, Ragù alla Bolognese and Nondairy Bechamel. The two recipes can be made several days ahead of time or earlier in the day. You also can cook the noodles ahead of time and refrigerate them between layers of waxed paper. Other convenient time-savers would be to use a ragù that you have made earlier and frozen and to make the bechamel sauce in the microwave.

Per serving: Calories 450, Protein 18 g, Soy Protein 11 g, Fat 15 g, Carbohydrates 55 g

15 to 18 uncooked lasagne noodles
1 recipe Ragù alla Bolognese (page 153)
1½ recipes (3 cups) thick Nondairy Bechamel (pages 96-97)
½ to 1 cup soy Parmesan

Cook the lasagne noodles in salted boiling water until al dente. Drain and rinse under cold water, then lay them flat between layers of waxed paper.

Preheat the oven to 350°F.

Oil a shallow 9 x 13-inch baking pan. Spread a thin layer of the ragù on the bottom of the pan. Cover with a layer of noodles, with the edges touching. Spread a layer of ragù over the noodles, then a layer of bechamel sauce, spreading it out evenly with the back of a spoon. Sprinkle with some of the soy Parmesan. Repeat the layers until everything is used up, ending with a layer of bechamel and soy Parmesan. Bake for 30 minutes.

Let the lasagne rest for 10 to 15 minutes before cutting it into squares.

❧ *Spinach Lasagne:* Mix 2 cups of Italian-Style Tofu Ricotta (page 95) or Quick Tofu Ricotta (page 93) with three 10-ounce packages of frozen chopped spinach, thawed and squeezed dry, or 3 pounds fresh spinach, cooked, squeezed dry, and chopped. Add 4 cloves garlic, crushed, ¼ teaspoon freshly grated nutmeg, and salt and freshly ground black pepper to taste. Add this as a layer after the ragù.

Spinach and "Cheese" Stuffed Crêpes

Yield: 6 servings

Serve these with a light tomato sauce or a medium bechamel or white sauce, pages 96-97, along with the soy Parmesan. Or you can layer the bechamel sauce over the tomato sauce for a really special dish.

Per serving: Calories 306, Protein 18 g, Soy Protein 12 g, Fat 9 g, Carbohydrates 36 g

Have ready:

3 cups tomato sauce or Nondairy Bechamel, pages 96-97

1 recipe Tofu Crêpes (pages 72-73)

2 onions, minced

1 tablespoon extra-virgin olive oil

2 pounds fresh spinach, well washed and drained, or two 10-ounce packages frozen chopped spinach

1½ cups crumbled medium-firm tofu

¼ cup soymilk

¼ teaspoon salt

4 to 6 tablespoons soy Parmesan

Salt, freshly ground black pepper, and nutmeg, to taste

> *Bright Idea:* You can also use other cooked greens instead of the spinach, use about twice as much ricotta and add a little Italian parsley for a "cheese" filling, or use the stuffing from the cannelloni on pages 146-47 to make a meat-style filling.

Sauté the onions in the olive oil in a nonstick skillet until they are soft and starting to brown. Add a tiny bit of water as needed, to keep them from sticking. Place the fresh spinach in boiling water until it is completely wilted, then drain, squeeze dry, and chop. If using frozen spinach, thaw it thoroughly and squeeze it as dry as possible; you can quick-thaw it by placing the whole carton in the microwave for 5 minutes.

Combine the crumbled tofu, soymilk, and ¼ teaspoon salt in a medium bowl. Add the cooked onions, spinach, soy Parmesan, and more salt, pepper, and nutmeg to taste. (It should be strongly seasoned.)

Preheat the oven to 425°F. Place a generous amount of filling down the center of each crêpe, and roll it up. Place the rolls in an oiled baking dish. Pour a little of the sauce you are using over the crêpes, sprinkle with soy Parmesan, and bake for 20 minutes. Serve with more sauce on the side.

Tofu Pot Pie

Yield: 6 servings

This recipe, adapted from The New Farm Vegetarian Cookbook *edited by Louise Hagler and Dorothy Bates, has remained a steady favorite of our family over the years. It is still the centerpiece of our vegetarian Thanksgiving and Christmas dinners, even when I serve a more elegant main dish as well.*

For holiday meals, I double the recipe and make it in a 14-inch cast-iron skillet. We serve it with mashed potatoes, cranberry sauce, and vegetable dishes. If you would like to make it more gourmet, you can use chanterelle mushrooms and add some chopped fresh herbs, such as savory, but we prefer it this way.

It may seem a bit of a production, but you could make the crust the day before, cook the tofu cubes when you have something else in oven, and make the filling a day or two before cooking. Then assemble the pie just before baking.

Per serving: Calories 342, Protein 17 g, Soy Protein 7 g, Fat 10 g, Carbohydrates 43 g

½ cup whole-wheat flour

2 tablespoons nutritional yeast flakes

1 teaspoon salt

½ teaspoon garlic granules

1 pound medium-firm tofu, cut into ½-inch cubes

1 large onion, chopped

2 medium carrots, peeled and diced

4 ounces fresh white or cremini mushrooms, sliced (1½ cups)

½ cup diced celery

¼ cup water

1½ cups frozen baby peas

2 tablespoons soy sauce

½ teaspoon garlic granules

1 recipe Brown Yeast Gravy (page 104) made with only 1 tablespoon soy sauce

One Low-Fat Pastry crust (pages 160-61)

Soymilk, to brush on top

Preheat the oven to 500°F. Mix the flour, nutritional yeast, salt, and garlic granules in a paper bag. Shake the tofu cubes in the bag until they are well-coated. Place the cubes on lightly oiled dark cookie sheets (dark sheets help brown faster), and bake for 7 to 10 minutes, or until golden on the bottom. Turn them over and bake 7 to 10 minutes more until golden all over. Remove from the oven and set aside.

Heat a large, lightly oiled or nonstick skillet over medium-high heat. Add the onion and steam-fry (see page 67) until they soften, adding a little water as necessary to keep from sticking. Add the carrots, mushrooms, celery, and water. Cover and cook for 10 minutes.

Add the peas, soy sauce, garlic granules, and the tofu cubes. If you are not baking the pie in the skillet, pour the mixture into a deep 10-inch casserole or pie pan, and stir in the Yeast Gravy.

Preheat the oven to 400°F.

Roll out the pie crust to fit the pan, and cover the tofu mixture with it. Cut decorative slits in the top, crimp the edges, and brush with soymilk. Place the pan on a 14-inch round pizza pan or a cookie sheet to catch any drips. Bake for 30 minutes. Serve hot.

For individual servings, you can make this in small pie pans or casserole dishes which can be frozen before baking.

Vegetarian Taco Filling

Yield: enough for 12 tacos or tostadas or 6 burritos

If you have some firm tofu in the freezer, some Red Chili Paste (page 109) in the refrigerator, and a package of taco shells, this deliciously spicy, kid-pleasing dinner won't take long. This also works for tostadas and burritos.

Per burrito: Calories 124, Protein 9 g, Soy Protein 9 g, Fat 7 g, Carbohydrates 4 g

1½ to 1¾ pounds firm tofu, frozen at least 48 hours,
   thawed, crumbled, and squeezed dry
¼ cup Red Chili Paste (page 109)
1 tablespoon extra-virgin olive oil
1 large onion, chopped
½ cup water or vegetarian broth (optional)

Mix the frozen tofu and Red Chili Paste in a bowl, combining well.

In a large nonstick skillet, heat the olive oil over medium-high heat. Add the onion and sauté until soft. Add the tofu-chili paste mixture, and cook over low heat for about 10 minutes, adding a little water or broth if it dries out too much.

Fill heated taco or tostada shells or whole-wheat tortillas for burritos, and add shredded lettuce or cabbage, a spicy tomato salsa, and Tofu Sour Cream (page 97). Cooked pinto or black beans or vegetarian refried beans are a good addition. You also can add some hash brown potatoes and grated nondairy cheese.

Pineapple Sweet and Sour

Yield: 6 servings

This restaurant favorite is a cinch to make at home. You have two low-fat crispy soy options to choose from.

Per serving: Calories 221, Protein 15 g, Soy Protein 14 g, Fat 0 g, Carbohydrates 39 g

1 large onion, cut into eighths

1 clove garlic, minced

1 teaspoon grated fresh gingerroot

One 19-ounce can unsweetened pineapple chunks with their juice

1 green bell pepper, seeded and cut into 1-inch squares

1 red bell pepper, seeded and cut into 1-inch squares

¼ cup cider vinegar or rice vinegar

⅓ cup light unbleached sugar or grade A light maple syrup

¼ cup ketchup

1 tablespoon soy sauce

2 tablespoons cornstarch or wheat starch dissolved in 2 tablespoons cold water

Choose 1 of the following:

2½ cups dry textured soy protein chunks

12 to 16 ounces Oven-Fried Tofu (page 110), cut in half or thirds

If you are using the textured soy chunks, reconstitute in 2½ cups boiling water, either soaking or simmering until tender. Drain well and pat dry. Roll in flour or cornstarch, and bake in single layers on dark cookies sheets at 500°F for about 7 minutes. (Dark cookie sheets brown foods better.) Then turn over and bake the other side for 5 to 7 minutes, or until golden all over

Bright Idea: Instead of soy protein chunks or oven-fried tofu, you can use 3 cups of commercial Japanese deep-fried tofu squares or triangles. (Cut the triangles in half.) This option is higher in fat, but very quick.

In a large, lightly oiled wok or heavy skillet, steam-fry (see page 67) the onion, garlic, and ginger over high heat, stirring constantly and adding drops of water if necessary to keep the vegetables from sticking. When the onion begins to become slightly translucent, add the pineapple, peppers, sugar, vinegar, ketchup, and soy sauce, and bring the mixture to a boil. Add the soy protein chunks or oven-fried tofu and dissolved cornstarch, and cook over high heat until the sauce thickens and the soy chunks or tofu are heated through, about 2 minutes. Serve immediately over rice.

Ragù alla Bolognese

This ragù is the traditional topping for tagliatelle and tortellini, but you can use it on any pasta, polenta, or gnocchi, or in Lasagne al Forno Bolognese (page 148). The toasted sesame oil used here is a good flavor substitute for the bacon traditionally added to the sauce.

Per ½ cup: Calories 135, Protein 3 g, Soy Protein 3 g, Fat 6 g, Carbohydrates 12 g

2 tablespoons extra-virgin olive oil

2 teaspoons toasted sesame oil

1 medium onion, minced

1 carrot, minced

1 stalk celery, minced

2 cloves garlic, minced

2 to 3 cups vegetarian hamburger crumbles or reconstituted beef-style textured soy granules

⅔ cup dry red or white wine, or ⅓ cup dry white wine and ⅓ cup marsala, dry sherry, or Madeira

1½ cups vegetarian broth

1½ cups chopped fresh, ripe plum tomatoes or canned, chopped plum tomatoes, drained and processed briefly in a food processor

1 teaspoon dried rosemary (optional)

4 to 5 fresh sage leaves, chopped

2 cups hot soymilk

Salt and freshly ground black pepper, to taste

In a medium-sized, heavy stockpot, heat the oils together over medium-high heat. Add the onion, carrot, celery, and garlic, and sauté until the vegetables are soft, stirring frequently. Add the hamburger crumbles and cook for a few minutes. Add the wine and cook over high heat until it has almost evaporated. Add the broth and cook over high heat until it reduces by at least half.

Add the tomatoes, sage, and rosemary, if desired, and cook for a few more minutes. Slowly stir in the heated soymilk, then reduce the heat and simmer, uncovered, for about 2 hours. Add salt and pepper to taste.

California Tamale Pie

Yield: 8 servings

If you like, you can make two 9-inch tamale pies and freeze one of them unbaked; then just thaw and bake it for a quick meal. You also could make individual tamale pies in small pie pans or casserole dishes, which also can be frozen..

Per serving: Calories 263, Protein 15 g, Soy Protein 10 g, Fat 0 g,
Carbohydrates 48 g

Filling:
2 large onions, chopped
2 cloves garlic, minced
2 tablespoons chili powder
1 teaspoon each dried oregano and ground cumin
5½ cups water
2 cups dry textured soy protein granules
2 cups frozen or canned corn kernels, drained
2 large green peppers, seeded and diced
Two 6-ounce cans tomato paste
¼ cup soy sauce
2 tablespoons unbleached sugar

½ teaspoon dried red chili pepper flakes (optional)
½ cup sliced pitted black California olives (optional)
1 to 2 cups cooked or canned pinto beans, drained (optional)
Salt, to taste
Cornmeal Topping:
1½ cups coarse yellow cornmeal
1½ cups cold water
1½ tablespoons vegetable broth powder
1 teaspoon salt
2½ cups boiling water
1 tablespoon extra-virgin olive oil or nondairy margarine (optional)

Lightly oil a large, heavy stockpot. Steam-fry the onions and garlic over medium heat (see page 67) until the onions are soft and starting to brown. Add the chili powder, oregano, and cumin, and cook for a few minutes. Add the remaining filling ingredients to the pan, and bring to a boil. Turn down and simmer, uncovered, while you make the cornmeal topping. Add salt to taste, but you probably won't need any.

Preheat the oven to 375°F.

In a large, heavy saucepan, mix the cornmeal with the cold water. Add the vegetable broth powder and salt, and then slowly stir in the remaining boiling water. Stir over high heat with a wooden spoon until it thickens. Turn the heat to low, and cook for 5 minutes.

To cook cornmeal topping in the microwave, mix 4 cups of cold water and the cornmeal, broth powder, and salt in a large microwave-proof bowl or 10-inch casserole. Microwave on high, uncovered, for 5 minutes.

Whisk and microwave for 3 minutes, then whisk and microwave 3 minutes more.

If you like, stir the optional olive oil or margarine into the cornmeal topping.

Pour the filling into a 9 x 13-inch pan or two 10-inch pie pans. Drop spoonfuls of the topping over the filling, then smooth them out as well as you can, patching any holes. If you wish, you can decorate the top with green or red bell pepper rings and grated nondairy cheese. Bake for 40 minutes.

Tofu Provençal

Yield: 4 servings

This is a fast and simple dish that is good enough for company. I prefer to use slices of extra-firm tofu that have been marinated in the Breast of Tofu marinade (see page 144) for more flavor, but the sauce here is tasty enough to use on plain tofu. We like this on steamed rice, but it's also delicious simply served with crusty bread to mop up the juices and a green salad on the side.

Per serving: Calories 166, Protein 8 g, Soy Protein 6 g, Fat 8 g, Carbohydrates 9 g

1 tablespoon extra-virgin olive oil

¾ pound extra-firm tofu or pressed tofu, cut into ¼-inch-thick slices

4 cloves garlic, minced

1 large onion, chopped

One 14-ounce can diced tomatoes and juice

1¼ cups vegetarian broth

⅓ cup dry white or dry red wine

⅓ cup fresh chopped basil

3 tablespoons chopped black olives, such as niçoise or kalamata

Salt and freshly ground black pepper, to taste

Heat the oil in a large nonstick skillet over medium-high heat. Sauté the tofu slices until brown on both sides. Add the garlic and onion, and sauté, stirring frequently, for a couple of minutes. Add the broth, tomatoes, and wine, and cook over high heat until the mixture cooks down and thickens. Add the basil, olives, and salt and pepper to taste. Serve immediately.

Tofu and Vegetable Oven-Broiled Stew

Yield: 6 to 8 servings

This delicious recipe, which has become a favorite for quick dinners, was developed first as a filling for bread. It was so good, and so quick and easy to make, that we have made it many times since, with several variations.

Per serving: Calories 120, Protein 5 g, Soy Protein 4 g, Fat 7 g, Carbohydrates 8 g

¾ to 1 pound uncooked, marinated Breast of Tofu, cut into cubes instead of slices (page 144)

2 carrots, peeled and thinly sliced on the diagonal or julienned

2 large onions, cut into ¼-inch slices

6 to 8 ounces fresh mushrooms (any kind), thickly sliced

2 stalks celery, diced

12 cloves garlic, sliced

2 tablespoons extra-virgin olive oil

2 teaspoons toasted sesame oil

1 cup Breast of Tofu marinade (page 144) or vegetarian broth

¼ cup chopped fresh Italian parsley

Salt and freshly ground black pepper, to taste

Optional:

Chunks of red or orange bell pepper

Sliced fennel

Juice of 2 lemons, or ½ cup dry white wine

1 to 2 tablespoons chopped fresh herbs, such as rosemary, sage, thyme, and basil

1 cup Easy Soy Cream (page 99) mixed with 2 teaspoons cornstarch

Preheat the broiler.

Place the tofu, vegetables, garlic, oils, and ½ cup of marinade or broth in two 9 x 13-inch pans. Place the pans 3 to 4 inches from the flame, and broil for about 10 minutes until the tops start to brown and scorch a little and the juices begin to evaporate. Add the rest of the broth and the lemon juice or wine, if using. Stir the mixture and place under the broiler again. When the tops begin to brown and scorch, add the parsley and any other herbs, if desired. Stir and continue broiling until the carrots are crisp-tender, the tofu is browned, and there are just enough pan juices to moisten the dish. You probably won't need salt because of the saltiness of the marinade or broth, but add salt and pepper to taste.

If you like, stir in the Easy Soy Cream and broil the mixture until the liquid has thickened a little, stirring the mixture well.

Serve with crusty bread, polenta, baked potatoes, plain rice, or broad eggless noodles.

Soy Bourguignone

Yield: 4 servings

This delicious French-inspired stew is a good way to try textured soy protein chunks. Serve it with crusty bread to mop up the gravy.

Per serving: Calories 292, Protein 14 g, Soy Protein 13 g, Fat 7 g, Carbohydrates 21 g

1 tablespoon extra-virgin olive oil

1 tablespoon toasted sesame oil

1½ cups unreconstituted textured soy protein chunks

Seasoned Flour (page 144)

2 onions, thinly sliced

3 cloves garlic, minced

¼ cup chopped celery

¼ cup chopped carrots

1 teaspoon unbleached sugar

1 cup vegetarian broth

1 cup dry red wine (can be nonalcoholic)

1 bay leaf

1 tablespoon tomato paste

1 teaspoon Marmite, yeast extract, or dark miso

½ teaspoon dried thyme

½ pound whole button mushrooms

¼ cup minced fresh parsley

Salt and freshly ground pepper, to taste

Reconstitute the textured soy chunks in 1½ cups boiling water, either soaking or simmering until tender. (See page 54.) Drain well and pat dry.

Heat the olive oil and sesame oil in a large, heavy pot over medium-high heat. Dredge the soy protein chunks in the seasoned flour, then sauté until brown. Remove from the pan and set aside. Add the onions to the pan, and sauté over medium heat until the onions start to soften, adding a little water as necessary to keep from sticking. Add the garlic, celery, carrots, and sugar. Continue cooking until the onions are soft and well browned. It is essential that the onions be well browned or caramelized, but not burned.

Add the soy protein to the pan, along with all the remaining ingredients, except the mushrooms, parsley, salt, and pepper. Cover and cook over low heat for 1 hour. Add the mushrooms and cook half an hour more. Just before serving, add the parsley and salt and pepper to taste. If the gravy is too thick, add a little more broth or wine. If the flavor does not seem meaty enough, add a little soy sauce instead of salt.

Chapter 12

Desserts

Although I don't advocate eating desserts every day, they give you another excellent opportunity to add soyfoods to your menus. Soymilk, tofu, and soy protein isolate powder can replace dairy products and some fat in your desserts while still giving you the satisfaction and mouth-feel of all those creamy, cheesy goodies that add fats, calories, and unwanted animal protein to your diet.

I use unbleached sugar because regular cane sugar is bleached with ashes made from cattle bones. (If you live east of the Rockies, you can purchase beet sugar, which is not bleached with animal products.) There are various types and brands of unbleached sugar on the market. Some are pale beige—this is what I refer to as *light unbleached sugar*. This can be used instead of white sugar in most recipes. Some look like brown sugar and is what I mean by *dark unbleached sugar*. You can use granulated sugar cane juice instead of dark unbleached sugar. If I don't specify light or dark, you can use either.

For ideas for baking with soy and substituting soy products for dairy products and eggs, see pages 61-64. You'll also find ideas there for lowering the fat in baked goods without compromising flavor and texture.

Finally, I am including some soy whipped toppings that my family likes, but if you are a fan of or occasionally use Cool-Whip or similar brands of whipped topping, try adding some soymilk to it, folding it in with a spatula. The soymilk makes it less dense and sweet and more like the texture of the real thing, besides adding soy's benefits to a product with little nutritional value.

Whipped Tofu Cream

Yield: 1¾ cups

This tastes very rich and decadent but is actually quite low in fat. It makes a great all-purpose nondairy whipped topping for desserts. You can vary the flavor with a tablespoon of liqueur, such as amaretto or Frangelico, or a dash of flavored extract. Keep in mind that tahini has a stronger flavor than other nut butters.

Per 2 tablespoons: Calories 40, Protein 2 g, Soy Protein 2 g, Fat 2 g, Carbohydrates 4 g

One 12.3-ounce package extra-firm silken tofu

2 to 4 tablespoons grade A light maple syrup, or to taste

2 tablespoons almond, cashew, or hazelnut butter or sesame tahini

Pinch of salt

Combine all the ingredients in a food processor or blender, adding more or less maple syrup to taste, until very smooth. Refrigerate for several hours before serving. This will keep refrigerated one week.

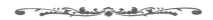

Sweet Thick Soy Pouring Cream

Yield: about ⅞ cup

This is a very smooth cream for beverages and desserts. It has a rich flavor and texture that belies its very low fat content. Coconut extract, an optional ingredient, doesn't make it taste like coconut but instead gives the cream a richer flavor. Using a nondairy milk other than soy will reduce the amount of soy flavor, as well.

Per 2 tablespoons: Calories 63, Protein 3 g, Soy Protein 3 g, Fat 1 g, Carbohydrates 10 g

½ cup plain rice milk or almond milk

½ cup extra-firm silken tofu

4 teaspoons grade A light maple syrup

Pinch of salt

1 tablespoon vegetable oil (optional)

¼ teaspoon coconut extract (optional)

Combine all the ingredients in a blender, and process until very smooth. (Be patient.) This can be refrigerated for several days. Stir gently before using.

Low-Fat Pastry

Yield: one 9-inch crust

Although this crust does contain fat, it has about half that of ordinary pastry, and it uses oil rather than hard fat. Divided into 8 servings, each piece with either a bottom or a top crust (not both) and a fat-free filling will contain 5 grams of fat. The pastry flour and soured soymilk make a tender crust that no one will guess is low-fat! (This recipe first appeared in the November 1994 issue of Vegetarian Times *magazine.)*

Per serving: Calories 98, Protein 2 g, Soy Protein 0 g, Fat 5 g, Carbohydrates 10 g

½ cup unbleached white flour

Scant ½ cup whole-wheat pastry flour

⅜ teaspoon salt

⅜ teaspoon baking powder

⅜ teaspoon sugar

3 tablespoons soymilk with ½ teaspoon lemon juice added

3 tablespoons oil (such as canola)

Note: If you have no whole-wheat pastry flour, use ½ cup regular whole-wheat flour and a scant ½ cup white pastry flour instead.

Mix the flours in a medium bowl with the salt, baking powder, and sugar. Whisk together the soured soymilk and oil in a cup until well blended. Pour this into the flour mixture, and mix gently with a fork until it holds together in a ball. (If it's too dry, sprinkle with a tiny bit of water.) If you have time, place the dough in a plastic bag and refrigerate it for an hour before rolling out. Roll out and bake as you would an ordinary crust, according to the particular recipe you are using.

To pre-bake an unfilled crust or bake "blind," preheat the oven to 425°F. Roll out the dough to fit a 9 or 10-inch tart or pie pan. Trim the top edge neatly. Prick the bottom and sides with a fork. Place a square of foil over the dough, and weight down with a layer of dried beans. Bake for 6 minutes. Remove the beans and foil, and bake 8 minutes more. Cool the pastry on a rack.

For a double crust pie: Use 1 cup unbleached flour, ⅞ cup whole-wheat pastry flour (or 1 cup regular whole-wheat flour and ⅞ cup white pastry flour), 6 tablespoons oil, 6 tablespoons soymilk curdled with 1 teaspoon lemon juice, and ¾ teaspoon each sugar, salt, and baking powder.

Microwave Option: Use a glass or ceramic pan, prick the pastry all over, and microwave on high for 6 to 7 minutes or until the pastry is opaque and the bottom is dry. (It will not brown.)

♦ *Savory Pies:* You can use olive oil and/or you can add ½ teaspoon curry powder, if you like.

♦ *Italian Sweet Pastry:* Use 2 tablespoons finely ground light unbleached sugar and add ½ teaspoon pure lemon extract and ¼ teaspoon pure vanilla extract. Do not use the microwave option for this variation.

Sweetened Condensed Soymilk

Yield: 1⅔ cups, equal to 1 commercial 14-ounce can

I devised this primarily to make Vietnamese Coffee (page 85), but it can be used in baking and candy-making instead of canned condensed dairy milk. It's fast to make and keeps in the refrigerator for several weeks.

Per 2 tablespoons: Calories 85, Protein 4 g, Soy Protein 4 g, Fat 0 g, Carbohydrates 15 g

1 cup light unbleached sugar

⅔ cup boiling water

6 tablespoons soymilk powder

5 tablespoons soy protein isolate powder

1 tablespoon melted nondairy margarine

Combine all the ingredients in a blender, and process until the sugar is dissolved and the mixture is thick. Pour into a clean jar, cover, and refrigerate. The milk thickens when chilled.

Panna Cotta

Yield: 8 servings

This rich molded pudding is a specialty of the Emiglia-Romagna region, which makes some of the richest dishes in Italy. Usually made of cream thickened with gelatin, panna cota is traditionally served by itself, but modern recipes often pair it with fruit or fruit sauce. This makes an excellent light dessert after an elegant company meal.

Per serving: Calories 124, Protein 5 g, Soy Protein 3 g, Fat 5 g, Carbohydrates 15 g

¾ teaspoon agar powder, or 1½ tablespoons agar flakes

2⅓ cups soymilk

One 12.3-ounce package extra-firm silken tofu

7 tablespoons light unbleached sugar

⅓ cup raw cashew pieces, ground

5 teaspoons each vanilla and fresh lemon juice

¾ teaspoon lemon extract or grated lemon zest (preferably organic)

¼ teaspoon salt

To cook the pudding on the stove top, soak the agar in the soymilk in a heavy saucepan while you proceed with the next step. To cook it in the microwave, soak the agar in the milk in a large microwave-proof bowl.

In a food processor or blender, process the tofu, sugar, ground cashews, vanilla, lemon juice, lemon extract or zest, and salt until very smooth—be patient!

Heat the milk and agar in the saucepan over high heat, stirring until it comes to a boil, then reduce the heat and simmer for 2 minutes. Or heat the milk and agar in the microwave on high for 2 minutes; stir, then cook on high for 2 more minutes.

Pour the hot milk mixture into the feeder tube of the food processor or the top of the blender while the motor is running. Mix well. Stop and stir down the bubbles.

Rinse 8 wide-bottom custard cups or molds with cold water, then pour the pudding into them. Chill until firm and cold. To serve, dip the bottoms of the molds in hot water for a few seconds to loosen, and unmold carefully on small dessert plates.

❧ *Crème Caramel:* Omit the lemon extract or lemon zest. Before making the pudding, combine 5 tablespoons unbleached sugar and 3 tablespoons water in a small saucepan. Simmer uncovered for 5 minutes until it thickens into a syrup. Divide the syrup evenly among the 8 custard cups, and rotate each cup to coat the bottom and sides. Pour the pudding on top, and proceed as directed. When unmolded, each pudding will have a coating of syrup on top.

❧ *Pumpkin Caramel Custard:* Omit the lemon extract or lemon zest. Replace ⅔ cup of the soymilk with ⅔ cup canned puréed pumpkin. Increase the amount of sugar to ½ cup plus 2 tablespoons total. Add ¼ teaspoon pumpkin pie spice or to taste. Use the syrup topping from Crème Caramel on the bottom of the facing page. Add 1 tablespoon minced candied ginger to the syrup, if you like.

❧ *Cappuccino Creams:* Omit the lemon zest or lemon extract. After making the Panna Cotta, pour half the mixture into a small bowl and stir in 1¾ tablespoons instant espresso powder. Keep the coffee mixture over heat just warm enough to keep it liquid. Pour the reserved (white) mixture evenly into the custard molds, and let it chill until firmed up a bit. Pour the coffee mixture over the white mixture. Chill and unmold as above. Decorate with crushed espresso beans, chocolate-covered espresso beans, grated nondairy semisweet chocolate, or one part unsweetened Dutch cocoa mixed with one part dark unbleached sugar.

❧ *Coconut Custard:* This is a great ending to both Asian and South American meals. Use only 2½ teaspoons vanilla and add 1 teaspoon coconut extract. Omit the lemon extract or lemon zest. Increase the amount of sugar to ½ cup plus 2 tablespoons total. Top with tropical fruits, such as pineapple, mango, or papaya. You may use the syrup topping from the Crème Caramel on the bottom of the facing page if you wish.

Sweet Ricotta Cream

This is delicious over fruit and other desserts or as an alternative to commercial nondairy whipped toppings.

In a blender or food processor, combine one batch of Italian-Style Tofu Ricotta (page 95) with ¼ cup grade A light maple syrup and 1 teaspoon vanilla. Mix until very smooth. (Be patient.)

Chocolate Bread Pudding

Yield: 6 servings

This is a low-fat treat that uses not only soy but leftover bread. Serve with your favorite nondairy whipped topping. A good brand of powdered egg replacer to use here is Ener-G Egg Replacer, available at most natural food stores or from the sources on page 184.

Per serving: Calories 191, Protein 7 g, Soy Protein 2 g, Fat 6 g, Carbohydrates 26 g

2 cups cubes of slightly stale Italian or French bread, crusts removed

2 cups soymilk

1 tablespoon powdered egg replacer (see the sources on page 61)

¼ cup water or cold strong coffee

2 teaspoons vanilla

2 tablespoons coffee, chocolate, orange, or nut liqueur (optional)

⅓ cup unsweetened Dutch cocoa

⅓ cup unbleached sugar

¼ teaspoon salt

¼ cup toasted chopped nuts

½ teaspoon cinnamon (optional)

In a medium bowl, soak the bread cubes in the soymilk for 10 minutes. Meanwhile, in a small, deep bowl, beat the egg replacer and water or coffee until it has the texture of softly beaten egg whites. Fold into the bread mixture along with the vanilla and liqueur, if using.

Preheat the oven to 375°F. In a small bowl, mix together the cocoa, sugar, salt, and cinnamon if using. Fold the dry ingredients into the bread mixture, mixing well. Pour the mixture into either a lightly greased 9-inch square or 7 x 11-inch baking pan, and bake for 45 minutes. Cool for at least a half hour before serving.

Chocolate Pudding

Yield: 4 servings

The ultimate comfort food! Use the coconut extract to add a richer flavor.

Per serving: Calories 143, Protein 4 g, Soy Protein 3 g, Fat 3 g, Carbohydrates 25 g

2 cups soymilk

⅓ cup unbleached sugar

¼ cup unsweetened Dutch cocoa

3 tablespoons cornstarch

1 to 2 tablespoons soy protein isolate powder (optional)

¼ teaspoon coconut extract (optional)

½ tablespoon instant coffee or coffee substitute (optional)

Pinch of salt

1 teaspoon vanilla

1 tablespoon Kahlua or other liqueur (optional)

Mix all the ingredients except the vanilla and liqueur, if using, in a blender or with a hand blender until smooth. Pour into a medium, heavy-bottomed saucepan. Stir the mixture constantly over high heat with a wooden spoon until it thickens and comes to a boil. Reduce the heat to low, cover, and cook 1 minute. Stir in the vanilla and optional liqueur.

Microwave method:

Cover a large microwave-safe bowl and microwave on high for 5 minutes. Whisk in the vanilla and liqueur, if using.

Pour into 4 pudding dishes or custard cups, cover, and refrigerate for several hours. If you don't want a skin on top, place plastic wrap right on the surface of the pudding.

Tofu Chocolate Mousse

Yield: 4 servings

This recipe has probably converted more people to tofu afficionados than any other recipe of mine. Try using orange or raspberry juice in place of the coffee.

Per serving: Calories 169, Protein 7 g, Soy Protein 6 g, Fat 3 g, Carbohydrates 28 g

½ cup unbleached sugar

3½ tablespoons strong coffee or espresso, coffee substitute, or water

4½ tablespoons unsweetened Dutch cocoa

One 12.3-ounce package firm or extra-firm silken tofu

1¼ teaspoons vanilla

Pinch of salt

1½ tablespoons rum, or coffee, chocolate, or other liqueur, or flavored Italian syrup for coffees (optional)

¼ teaspoon cinnamon (optional)

Mix the sugar and coffee or water in a small saucepan, and stir over high heat until dissolved. Stir in the cocoa until a paste forms. Place this in a food processor or blender with the tofu, vanilla, salt, and the liqueur and cinnamon, if using, and process until very smooth. Pour into 4 pudding dishes or goblets, cover, and chill for several hours.

For a richer version or a rich pie filling, add ½ cup melted semisweet nondairy chocolate chips to the processed mixture.

❧ *Frozen Chocolate Tofulato:* Double the recipe for the basic version, and add 1 cup melted semisweet nondairy chocolate chips and ½ cup plus 2 tablespoons soymilk. Chill. Follow the directions for your ice cream maker.

❧ *Fudgesicles:* Omit the coffee and liqueur, and use 6 tablespoons water. Use only 3 tablespoons cocoa. Freeze the mixture in popsicle molds.

❧ *Chocolate Tofu Cream Pie:* Double the recipe for the basic version, using extra-firm silken tofu, and add 1 cup melted semisweet nondairy chocolate chips. Spread the mixture in a prebaked, cooled 9-inch Low-Fat Pastry Crust (pages 160-61) or the Crumb Crust from the Cheesecake recipe (page 172). Chill thoroughly and top with your favorite nondairy whipped topping (page 158), Whipped Tofu Cream (page 159), or Sweet Ricotta Cream (page 163). For Chocolate-Banana Cream Pie, place sliced bananas over the crust, spread on half the mousse, add another layer of bananas, and then spread on the remaining mousse.

Chocolate-Peanut Butter Tofu Pie

Yield: 8 to 10 servings

This is not a low-fat dessert, but it is considerably lower in fat than similar pies that use melted chocolate. It's a great dessert for those times when you want something really rich. If you are allergic to peanuts, use roasted almond or cashew butter, or any other nut butter that you prefer.

Per serving: Calories 181, Protein 8 g, Soy Protein 3 g, Fat 8 g, Carbohydrates 19 g

One baked and cooled 8- or 9-inch Low-Fat Pastry Crust (pages 160-61)

Filling:

One 12.3-ounce package extra-firm silken tofu

2½ tablespoons water

½ cup plus 1½ tablespoons unbleached sugar

½ cup plus 1½ tablespoons unsweetened Dutch cocoa

1¼ teaspoons vanilla

⅛ teaspoon salt

Scant ½ cup smooth or crunchy natural peanut butter

2 tablespoons chopped roasted peanuts

Place all of the filling ingredients in a food processor or blender, and process until very smooth. Pour into the cooled crust, and smooth the top. Garnish the top with the roasted peanuts. Chill and serve with Whipped Tofu Cream (page 159), Sweet Ricotta Cream (page 163), or your favorite nondairy whipped topping. (See the note on page 158.)

Millennium Mudpie Cake

Yield: one 8-inch square cake or one 9- or 10-inch round cake (8 servings)

This is a new version of a wartime eggless cake that became very popular in the 1950s and '60s—also called Wacky Cake or Crazy Cake because it was mixed right in the pan. My kids loved making it and eating it. I've changed the original version, which used water, to make it soy-rich and cut the oil in half. Also, because it's a thin batter and coarse unbleached sugar often sinks to the bottom, I mix the sugar with the liquid ingredients in this version to avoid that.

It's easy, chocolaty, and tender, so we often use it as a layer cake (double or triple the recipe to make layers), a sheet cake (double the recipe and bake in two 9-inch round pans or a 9 x 13-inch pan), or for cupcakes (one recipe makes about 9). Try it with Chocolate-Soy Ganache on the next page, Broiled Coconut Frosting (see the Bright Idea below), or any other favorite icing. Nonchocolate variations can be used for upside-down cakes, fruit-topped cakes, and so forth.

Per serving: Calories 230, Protein 5 g, Soy Protein 2 g, Fat 6 g, Carbohydrates 39 g

Dry Mix:

1¼ cups pastry flour

⅓ cup unsweetened Dutch cocoa

2 tablespoons soy protein isolate powder

1 teaspoon baking soda

¼ teaspoon salt

Liquid Mix:

1 cup unbleached sugar

1 cup plus 3 tablespoons soymilk

3 tablespoons oil

1 tablespoon vinegar

1½ teaspoons vanilla

Preheat the oven to 350°F.

Whisk the dry mix ingredients together in a medium bowl. Combine the liquid mix ingredients in a blender until smooth, then pour into the dry ingredients and mix briefly—do not beat. Pour the batter into a lightly oiled 8-inch square or 9-inch round cake pan. Bake for 25 minutes, or until a toothpick inserted in the center comes out clean. Thoroughly cool on a rack before eating. Serve right from the pan, or gently loosen and invert on a plate. Frost as desired, or serve with nondairy whipped topping and fruit.

Bright Idea: My kids used to love this with Broiled Coconut Frosting, which makes it taste a bit like a German chocolate cake. To make the frosting, mix together ⅓ cup dark unbleached sugar, 2 tablespoons soymilk, ¾ cup unsweetened coconut flakes, and ½ cup chopped nuts, if desired. Spread over the cooled cake. Place the cake 3 to 4 inches below the oven broiler, and broil until bubbly and lightly browned. Watch carefully or it will burn!

❧ *White Wacky Cake:* This can be used for a cottage pudding with a fruit sauce, stewed fruit, or any sweet sauce; for upside-down cake; for a layer cake; or a cake sliced horizontally in half with jam spread between the layers. It's also good with a chocolate icing or ganache. Omit the cocoa and use a total of 1½ cups pastry flour. Use only ½ to ¾ cup light unbleached sugar, and use lemon juice instead of vinegar. Use only 1 teaspoon vanilla. You also can add ½ teaspoon of lemon, almond, coconut, or orange extract.

❧ *Queen Elizabeth Cake:* This is a favorite Canadian recipe. Add 1 cup chopped pitted dates to the White Wacky Cake version, and top the cooled cake with Broiled Coconut Frosting. (See the Bright Idea on the facing page.)

❧ *Spice Cake:* Use dark unbleached sugar in the White Wacky Cake version. Add ½ teaspoon cinnamon, ½ teaspoon ground allspice, and ¼ teaspoon freshly grated nutmeg.

❧ *Lemon Cake:* Omit the vanilla from the White Wacky Cake version. Use 4 tablespoons fresh lemon juice, and omit the 3 tablespoons soymilk. Add the grated zest of one lemon, preferably organic. If you like, add 2 to 4 tablespoons poppy seeds.

❧ *Orange Cake:* Add the grated zest of one orange, and ¾ cup dried currants or 2 to 4 tablespoons poppy seeds to the White Wacky Cake version. Omit the 3 tablespoons soymilk and lemon juice, and use ¼ cup orange juice. Top the warm cake with ½ cup orange marmalade melted with 1 teaspoon orange juice.

Chocolate-Soy Ganache

A ganache is a rich, fudgy chocolate icing that firms up when cooled. Process 6 ounces (1 cup) good-quality, dairy-free chocolate chips in a food processor until finely chopped. Whip ½ cup soymilk and ⅓ cup extra-firm silken tofu in a blender until very smooth. Heat the mixture in the top of a double boiler over simmering water until almost to the boiling point. Pour into the feed tube of the processor, and process until smooth. Scrape the mixture into a mixing bowl, and refrigerate just until it is completely cooled, but not chilled. Whip in 1 teaspoon vanilla, or 1 tablespoon liqueur of choice, and allow to chill for several hours, or until firm enough to use as a frosting. To soften, leave at room temperature until it is as soft as you like it. It will keep in the refrigerator for a couple of months.

French Strawberry Pie

Yield: 8 servings

This has to be everybody's favorite during strawberry season. Of course, if you grow ever-bearing strawberries, you can eat it all summer!

Per serving: Calories 166, Protein 2 g, Soy Protein 1 g, Fat 2 g, Carbohydrates 34 g
(without crust)

One 9-inch Low-Fat Pastry Crust, prebaked unfilled and cooled (pages 160-61)

Filling:

½ 12.3-ounce box extra-firm silken tofu, drained

2½ tablespoons raw cashew pieces, finely ground

1½ tablespoons lemon juice

¼ teaspoon salt

1½ tablespoons grade A light maple syrup

½ teaspoon vanilla

Glaze:

1 cup red currant jelly

¼ cup fresh lemon juice

Fruit:

2 pints fresh ripe strawberries

Garnish:

Whipped Tofu Cream (page 159), Sweet Ricotta Cream (page 163), or other favorite nondairy whipped topping

Several hours before serving, process the silken tofu, ground cashew pieces, 1½ tablespoons of lemon juice, salt, maple syrup, and vanilla in a blender or food processor until very smooth. You may have to stop the machine and scrape the sides with a spatula once or twice. Spread the mixture carefully on the bottom of the pie shell.

In a saucepan over high heat, melt the jelly with the ¼ cup lemon juice. Remove from the heat and let it cool until it is like a thick sauce.

Wash, pat dry, and trim the berries. Choose ones that are large, ripe, evenly red, and arrange them, bottoms-up, in the pie shell. If you have extras, you can slice and arrange them around the whole berries.

Drizzle the almost-cooled jelly mixture over the berries, coating them equally. Chill for a few hours before serving, but serve the same day. Garnish the pie with the whipped topping of your choice

Lemon Tofu Pie

Yield: 8 servings

This delicious, creamy pie is so easy to make that I'm sure it will become a year-round favorite.

Per serving: Calories 122, Protein 4 g, Soy Protein 4 g, Fat 2 g, Carbohydrates 21 g

One 9-inch Low-Fat Pastry Crust, prebaked for 5 minutes and cooled (pages 160-61)

Filling:

1 pound medium-firm tofu

¾ cup light unbleached sugar

½ cup fresh lemon juice

2 tablespoons cornstarch or wheat starch

Grated zest of 1 large lemon (preferably organic), or 2 teaspoons lemon extract

Preheat the oven to 350°F.

Combine all the filling ingredients in a blender or food processor until very smooth. Pour into the crust and bake for 35 minutes. Cool the pie on a rack, then refrigerate until serving time.

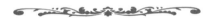

Lemon Cream

Yield: about 1¾ cups

This delicious cream can be used as a pudding or a topping for fruit or cake.

Per serving: Calories 34, Protein 2 g, Soy Protein 2 g, Fat 1 g, Carbohydrates 5 g

One 12.3-ounce package extra-firm silken tofu, crumbled

⅓ cup grade A light maple syrup

3 tablespoons fresh lemon juice

1 tablespoon grated lemon zest (preferably organic)

Combine all the ingredients in a blender, and process until very smooth. Chill in a covered container.

❦ *Lemon-Ginger Cream*: Fold in ¼ cup finely minced crystallized ginger.

Easy Tofu-Cashew Cheesecake

Yield: One 8-inch cheesecake (8 servings)

This is a small cheesecake for the simple reason that we usually overeat the big, thick ones; you are supposed to eat just a small slice of those, but who ever does? This tofu cheesecake is relatively low in fat but is still creamy and rich, and very easy to make. We thought it the best tofu cheesecake we'd ever tasted, and the fat-free graham cracker crust is excellent. The recipe may be doubled for an 8-inch springform pan. In this case, bake it for 50 to 60 minutes.

Per serving: Calories 221, Protein 4 g, Soy Protein 3 g, Fat 5 g, Carbohydrates 40 g

Crumb Crust:
¾ cup graham cracker crumbs
3 tablespoons light corn syrup

Filling:
One 12.3-ounce package extra-firm silken tofu
⅓ cup raw cashew pieces, finely ground
6 tablespoons unbleached sugar
Juice of one large lemon (about 5 tablespoons)
Finely grated zest of ½ large lemon (preferably organic)
1 tablespoon cornstarch
¼ teaspoon vanilla
¼ teaspoon salt

Optional Creamy Topping:
1 cup Tofu Sour Cream (page 97)
½ tablespoon light unbleached sugar
½ teaspoon vanilla

Fruit Preserve Topping:
½ cup low-sugar or fruit-sweetened fruit preserves
½ tablespoon lemon juice

Preheat the oven to 350°F.

Mix the graham cracker crumbs with the corn syrup, and press onto the bottom and sides of a lightly oiled 8-inch pie pan.

Place the filling ingredients in a food processor or blender, and combine until very smooth. (Be patient.) Pour into the crust and bake for 25 to 35 minutes until the filling is set and slightly cracked around the edges. Cool on a rack, then refrigerate for about 4 hours before serving.

If you are using the optional creamy topping, combine the ingredients in a blender or food processor or with a hand blender until smooth. Spread over the chilled cheesecake before you add the fruit preserve topping, or use instead of the fruit topping. For the fruit preserve topping, melt the preserves with the lemon juice in a small saucepan, then spread over the top of the cheesecake.

❧ *Lemon Cheesecake:* Use Lemon Cream (page 171) as the topping instead of the creamy topping and the fruit topping.

❧ *Espresso Cheesecake:* For the crust, use chocolate-wafer crumbs instead of graham cracker crumbs. For the filling, use only 1½ table-spoons lemon juice, omit the lemon zest, increase the vanilla to ½ tea-spoon, and add 3 tablespoons Kahlua and ¾ tablespoon instant espresso powder. If the mixture doesn't seem sweet enough, add about 2 table-spoons more sugar. Top the cooled cheesecake with Chocolate-Soy Ganache (page 169) while the ganache is still hot, and sprinkle with a few toasted almonds or hazelnuts. Chill for several hours.

❧ *Irish Coffee Cheesecake:* Follow the instructions for Espresso Cheesecake (above), but use Irish whiskey instead of Kahlua. Omit the Chocolate-Soy Ganache topping, and use Whipped Tofu Cream (page 159) instead.

❧ *Amaretto Cheesecake:* Use only 1½ tablespoons lemon juice, omit the lemon zest and vanilla, and add 3 tablespoons amaretto and ¼ tea-spoon pure almond extract. For the topping, mix 1 cup Tofu Sour Cream (page 97) with 1 tablespoon unbleached sugar, ¼ teaspoon vanilla, and ½ tablespoon amaretto. Sprinkle with ¼ cup toasted almonds.

❧ *Chocolate Cheesecake:* For the filling, omit the cornstarch and lemon zest. Use ½ cup plus 1 tablespoon unbleached sugar, 1½ table-spoons lemon juice, and ½ teaspoon vanilla. Add 2 tablespoons unsweet-ened Dutch cocoa and 3 tablespoons chocolate, coffee, almond, orange, or hazelnut liqueur. If you like, stir in 1 cup semisweet, nondairy mini-chocolate chips or chopped chocolate to the batter after blending. Use a topping of 1 cup Tofu Sour Cream (page 97) mixed with 1 tablespoon unbleached sugar, ½ tablespoon of liqueur, and ¼ teaspoon vanilla. Sprinkle the top with nondairy semisweet chocolate shavings.

❧ *Chocolate-Mint Cheesecake:* This variation—a great one for Christmas—was suggested by my good friend Holly Walker. For the crust, use chocolate-wafer crumbs instead of graham cracker crumbs. For the filling, use only 1½ tablespoons of lemon juice, and omit the lemon zest. Stir 1 cup of nondairy, semisweet minichocolate chips into the blended fill-ing before pouring it into the crust. After baking and cooling the cheese-cake, pour about ½ recipe of Chocolate-Soy Ganache (page 169), to which you have added ½ teaspoon peppermint extract, over the top of it, while the ganache is still warm. Spread evenly over the top, and chill for sev-eral hours.

❧ *Fresh Fruit Cheesecake:* Top the original cooled cheesecake, (with or without the Tofu Sour Cream Topping) with sliced fresh fruit of your choice in a decorative, overlapping design. Melt ¼ cup of apple jelly with ½ tablespoon lemon juice until bubbly. Paint the fruit with the jelly, using a pastry brush. You can also use red currant jelly on red fruits, or fruit-sweetened orange marmalade on orange slices. Chill for several hours.

Pumpkin Cheesecake

Yield: One 8-inch cheesecake (8 servings)

Per serving: Calories 197, Protein 4 g, Soy Protein 3 g, Fat 5 g, Carbohydrates 34 g

Have ready:
Crumb crust, page 172, using
   gingersnap crumbs instead of
   graham cracker crumbs
Filling:
One 12.3-ounce package extra-firm
   silken tofu
⅓ cup cashew pieces, finely ground
6 tablespoons dark unbleached
   sugar
6 tablespoons light unbleached
   sugar
1½ tablespoons lemon juice
2 tablespoons cornstarch
1 cup packed canned pumpkin
¾ teaspoon pumpkin pie spice

Preheat the oven to 350°F.

Place the filling ingredients in a food processor or blender, and combine until very smooth. (Be patient.) Pour into the crust and bake for 25 to 35 minutes until the filling is set and slightly cracked around the edges. Cool on a rack, then refrigerate for about 4 hours before serving.

Top with a nondairy whipped topping of your choice (see the note on page 158) or Whipped Tofu Cream (page 159).

Tofu-Cashew Cream Cheese Frosting

Yield: 2½ cups (enough for a 2- or 3-layer cake)

Creamy, rich-tasting, not-too-sweet—the perfect icing for celebration cakes.

Per 2 tablespoons: Calories 62, Protein 3 g, Soy Protein 2 g, Fat 2 g, Carbohydrates 6 g

Two 12.3-ounce packages extra-firm silken tofu

⅔ cup raw cashew pieces, finely ground

⅓ cup light grade A maple syrup

3 tablespoons plus 1 teaspoon lemon juice

1¼ teaspoons vanilla

½ teaspoon salt

Crumble the tofu into a clean tea towel, then gather up the ends. Twist and squeeze repeatedly until the tofu is as dry as possible. Blend all of the ingredients in a food processor (or in 2 batches in a blender) until very smooth. Refrigerate while you make the cake. Check the frosting when you take the cake out of the oven. If it is too firm to spread, leave it at room temperature while the cake cools. Refrigerate the frosted cake.

❧ Banana-Nut Cream Cheese Frosting: Add 1 small ripe mashed banana and ¼ cup minced toasted walnuts, pecans, or unsweetened coconut flakes.

❧ Lemon Cream Cheese Frosting: Use only 1 teaspoon vanilla, and add ¼ cup lemon juice and 1 tablespoon grated lemon zest (preferably organic).

Easy Fruit Tofulato

Yield: about 3½ to 4 cups

This frozen soy yogurt is easy, light, and delicious, and you can use any fruit, from berries, to peaches, to mangoes. If you use frozen fruit, measure by weight or by volume while it's frozen, and then let it thaw out before puréeing. Using the optional liqueur will prevent the gelato from freezing rock-hard, as well as add flavor; the optional vegetable oil will make the gelato richer. You'll need an ice cream maker for this recipe; one of those inexpensive ones with the metal insert that you freeze (like a Donvier) works just fine.

Per ¾ cup: Calories 193, Protein 7 g, Soy Protein 6 g, Fat 4 g, Carbohydrates 32 g

1½ cups lightly packed fresh berries or pitted, peeled, chopped fruit (see note above for frozen fruit)

1 pound medium-firm tofu plus ½ cup water, orange juice or other fruit juice, or two 12.3-ounce packages silken tofu, or 2 ½ cups plain soy yogurt (commercial or page 86)

About ¾ cup light unbleached sugar or grade A light maple syrup (use less if fruit is very sweet)

3 tablespoons fresh lemon juice

2 teaspoons vanilla, or 1 teaspoon vanilla plus 1 teaspoon orange, lemon, or other pure extract

Pinch of salt

Optional:

2 to 3 tablespoons vodka, rum, orange, almond, or other appropriate fruit liqueur or brandy

2 to 3 tablespoons neutral-tasting vegetable oil, such as canola

Purée the fresh or thawed frozen fruit in a blender or food processor; set aside.

Place the remaining the ingredients in a blender, and process until very smooth. Add the puréed fruit and blend well again. Pour the mixture into a covered container, and chill thoroughly before freezing in an ice cream maker according to the manufacturer's directions.

Scoop the tofulato into a quart plastic container; cover and freeze for a couple of hours before serving.

♦ *Piña Colada Tofulato:* Use an 8-ounce can of crushed unsweetened pineapple for the fruit; use 2 to 3 tablespoons dark rum, 1 teaspoon vanilla, and 1 teaspoon coconut extract. Top each serving with toasted coconut flakes.

Southern Peach Tofulato: Use fresh or frozen ripe peaches for the fruit, and use 2 to 3 tablespoons bourbon. Top each serving with chopped toasted pecans.

Italian Peach-Amaretto Tofulato: Make as for Southern Peach Tofulato, but use amaretto instead of bourbon and top each serving with chopped toasted almonds.

Easy Chocolate Soy Gelato

Yield: about 3 cups

This dessert tastes so rich and intense that it's hard to believe that it is low in fat. The soy protein makes the mixture very creamy and rich-tasting. Only for confirmed chocolate lovers! You need an ice cream maker for this recipe. Be sure to use only unsweetened dark or Dutch cocoa, which has the richest, deepest flavor without the fat.

Per ¾ cup: Calories 295, Protein 10 g, Soy Protein 8 g, Fat 3 g, Carbohydrates 52 g

1 cup water

1 cup unbleached sugar

¼ to ½ cup unsweetened Dutch cocoa, depending on how intense a chocolate flavor you want

1½ cups soymilk

⅓ cup soy protein isolate powder

2 tablespoons coffee, almond, hazelnut, or orange liqueur

1 tablespoon grated orange zest (preferably organic; optional)

In a medium stainless-steel saucepan over high heat, dissolve the sugar in the water, stirring constantly. Whisk in the cocoa powder over low heat, and continue to whisk it for a couple of minutes until it is completely smooth. Pour the mixture into a blender with the remaining ingredients, and process until smooth. Chill the mixture, then freeze in an ice cream maker according to the manufacturer's directions.

If you don't use liqueur, add ¼ teaspoon powdered agar or 1½ teaspoons agar flakes, soaked in the water for a few minutes, and then cooked with the sugar mixture. This keeps the gelato from becoming rock-hard. For more flavor, use strong coffee or orange juice instead of the water.

Bibliography

I don't necessarily agree with all of the nutritional advice in these resources, but they contain helpful, up-to-date information on a variety of subjects including nutrition, exercise, and health options.

Books

Andes, Karen. *A Woman's Book of Power: Using Dance to Cultivate Energy and Health in Mind, Body, and Spirit.* New York: Berkley Publishing Group, 1998. An excellent book from a personal trainer and author of *The Woman's Book of Strength*; strong bellydance overtones, but accessible to everyone.

Barnard, Neal M.D. *Eat Right to Live Longer.* New York: Harmony Books, 1995.

Cooper, Robert K., and Leslie L. Cooper. *Low-Fat Living.* Emmaus, Pa.: Rodale Press, 1996.

Epstein, Diane, and Kathleen Thompson. *Feeding on Dreams: Why America's Diet Industry Doesn't Work and What Will Work for You.* New York and Toronto: Macmillan Publishing Co., 1994. This is an excellent book for chronic dieters and women who have or have had eating disorders. It not only gives excellent practical advice about eating and exercising healthfully, planning a program that you can live with, and being realistic about your expectations and goals, but offers help to change the way you think about your body, about food, and about taking control of your life. Highly recommended!

Golbitz, Peter. *Tofu and Soyfoods Cookery: Delicious Soyfoods for a Healthy Life.* Summertown, Tenn.: Book Publishing Co., 1998. This book contains an extensive list of addresses, phone and fax numbers, e-mail addresses, and website addresses for U.S. and Canadian soyfood companies. Recipes by Louise Hagler, Dorothy R. Bates, Barb Bloomfield, Judy Brown, and Bryanna Clark Grogan.

Gray, Timothy J. D.O. *Back Works.* Seattle, Wash.: BookPartners, Inc., 1993. One of the most practical books I've found on how to prevent back pain and injury, and what to do if you have back pain. For more information you can contact the publisher at P.O. Box 19732, Seattle, WA, 98109

Greene, Bob, and Oprah Winfrey. *Make the Connection.* New York: Hyperion, 1996. A very inspiring book for chronic dieters.

Grogan, Bryanna Clark. *The Almost No-Fat Cookbook: Everyday Vegetarian Recipes*. Summertown, Tenn: Book Publishing Co., 1994.

———*The Almost No-Fat Holiday Cookbook: Festive Vegetarian Recipes*. Summertown, Tenn: Book Publishing Co., 1995.

———*20 Minutes to Dinner: Quick, Low-Fat, Low-Calorie Vegetarian Meals*. Summertown, Tenn: Book Publishing Co., 1997.

———*Nonna's Italian Kitchen: Delicious Homestyle Vegan Cuisine*. Summertown, Tenn: Book Publishing Co., 1998

Hagler, Louise. *Soyfoods Cookery: Your Road to Better Health*. Summertown, Tenn.: Book Publishing Co., 1996. See also her classic *Tofu Cookery*, and *The New Farm Vegetarian Cookbook*, which Hagler edited, published by the same company.

Jacobowitz, Ruth S. *150 Most-Asked Questions About Osteoporosis: What Women Really Want to Know*. New York: Hearst Books, 1993.

Kradjian, Robert M.D. *Save Yourself from Breast Cancer: Life Choices That Can Help You Reduce the Odds*. New York: Berkeley Books, 1994.

Lark, Susan M.D. *The Menopause Self Help Book, rev. ed.* Berkeley: Celestial Arts, 1990.

Laux, Marcus N.D., and Christine Conrad. *Natural Woman, Natural Menopause*. New York: HarperCollins, 1997. An excellent book which contains information on natural progestorone creams, natural estrogen therapies, herbs, diet, exercise, strength training, PMS relief, product sources, testing sources, and addresses of mail-order pharmacies that compound natural estrogens for you.

Melina, Vesanto; Brenda Davis; and Victoria Harrison. *Becoming Vegetarian: The Complete Guide to Adopting a Healthy Vegetarian Diet, rev. ed.* Summertown, Tenn.: Book Publishing Co., 1997. Written by three registered dieticians.

Messina, Mark and Virginia Messina. *The Simple Soybean and Your Health*. Garden City, N.Y.: Avery 1994.

Messina, Virginia and Mark Messina. *The Vegetarian Way*. New York: Crown, 1996. A complete vegetarian nutrition book by a registered dietician with a master's degree in public health nutrition and a doctor of nutrition who is one of the foremost authorities on soy. (The Messinas' internet site, "Nutrition Matters," is at: www.olympus.net/messina/)

Mindell, Earl. *Earl Mindell's Soy Miracle*. New York: Simon & Schuster, Fireside, 1995.

Nelson, Miriam E. *Stong Women Stay Slim*. New York: Bantam, 1998.
————*Strong Women Stay Young*. New York: Bantam, 1997.

Robbins, John. *Diet for a New America*. Walpole, N. H.: Stillpoint Publishing, 1987. A classic.

Vedral, Joyce L. *Bone-Building Body-Shaping Workout*. New York: Simon & Schuster, Fireside, 1998.

————*Bottoms Up!*. New York: Warner, 1993

————*Definition*. New York: Warner, 1995. The book that started me out with weight training;

————*The Fat-Burning Workout*. New York: Warner, 1991

————*Top Shape*. New York: Warner, 1995. For men

————*Weight Training Made Easy*. New York: Warner, 1997.

Waterhouse, Debra. *Outsmarting the Midlife Fat Cell*. New York: Hyperion, 1998.

Wharton, Jim, and Phil Wharton. *The Whartons' Stretch Book*. New York: Times Books, 1996. How to stretch properly for maximum flexibility, whether you are an athlete or just trying to keep fit.

Winter, Ruth. *Super Soy: The Miracle Bean*. New York: Crown, 1996.

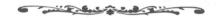

Websites

Menopause and women's health sites:
    www.thai-menopause.th.com/
    users.aol.com/mdlfwoman/info.htm
    www.healthy.net/clinic/dandc/menopaus/index.html
    inform.umd.edu:86/Educational_Resources/
    moose.uvm.edu/~mbilz/index.html
    www.cfe.cornell.edu/bcerf/
    hre.com/totalhealth/memopse.html

Vegetarian links:

    www.excite.com/lifestyle/food-and-drink/vegetarianism/

    hippy.com/veggie.htm

    www.vegetariancentral.org/

    dinnercoop.cs.cmu.edu/dinnercoop/special/vegetarian.html

    www/vegan.com/pages/links.html

    www.katsden.com/webster/veg.html

Other Sites:

American Soybean Association: www.oilseeds.org/asa/

Animal Rights Resource Site: //arrs.envirolink.org/index.html

BioFitness Systems, Inc.: www.biofitness.com: A website that gives a free accurate reading of your body fat and lean muscle percentages.

Book Publishing Company: www.bookpubco.com: Many excellent books on vegetarian cooking and vegetarian diet and nutrition.

Cooking Light magazine: www.cookinglight.com

Handilinks to Menopause: www/ahandyguide.com/cat1/m/m394.htm

International Vegetarian Union: www.ivu.org/

Menotimes: web.aimnet.com~hyperion/meno/monotimes.index.htm/

North American Vegetarian Society: www.cyberveg.org/navs/

The No Milk Page: wwww.panix.com/~nomilk/

Nutrition Action Newsletter, Center for Science in the Public Interest: www.cspinet.org

Nutritional Navigator: navigator.tufts.edu.

PETA (People for the Ethical Treatment of Animals): www.envirolink.org/arrs/peta/

Prevention magazine: www.healthyideas.com: This magazine pushes ERT and dairy products too much for my liking, but has some good articles about exercise and other aspects of health.

Shape magazine: www.fitnessonline.com/livingfit:
Website tailored for women over 35

Shape-Up America!: www.shapeup-org.

Soy Goodness Home Page: www2.ani.net/home3/health

Soy Links: trfn.clpgh.org/Lifestyle/cooking/soya.html

Soyatech, Inc.: www.soyatech.com

Toronto Vegetarian Association: www.veg.on.ca/

United Soybean Board: www.talksoy.com

Vegan Action: www.vegan.com/

The Vegan Page: members.aol.com/docvegan/

Vegan Society of UK: www.vegansociety.com

Vegetarian Pages: www.es.rochester.edu/u/sarukkai/veggie2.html

Vegetarian Recipe Directory: www/vegweb.com/food/

Vegetarian Recipes Sites: A List:
    www.cyber-kitchen.com/pgvegtar.htm

Vegetarian Resource Group: www.vrg.org/

Vegetarian Society of UK: www.vegsoc.org

Vegetarian Times magazine: www.vegetariantimes.com

Veggies Unite: www.envirolink.org/orgs/vegweb/

Very Vegetarian Sites: www.cyber-kitchen.com/pgvegtar.ontm

Walking magazine: www.walkingmag.com

World Guide to Vegetarianism: www.veg.org/veg/Guide/

www.joyofsoy.com: lots of soy links

www.soymilkmaker.com: a home soymilk maker you can purchase

Other Resources

United Soybean Hotline: 1-800-825-5769
 Soy recipes, health and agricultural information.
Vegetarian Voice, the magazine of the North American Vegetarian
 Society (Box 72, Dolgeville, NY, 13329)

Sources for Ingredients

Soy Parmesan

Soymage 100% Nondairy, Casein-free Grated Parmesan Cheese Alternative
 (called "Grated Tofu" in Canada),
Soymage Soychunk "Italian Flavor" vegan mozzarella cheese substitute:
 You'll probably want to take advantage of the substantial savings you can
 make by buying these products in bulk. They freeze well or you could order
 them through your co-op or food buying group and share a case with several people.
  To find a distributor to buy from in bulk or a health food store which
 carries these products in your area of the U.S., contact the manufacturer:
 Galaxy/SoyCo Foods
 1-800-441-9419, cxt. 322;
 e-mail galxsales@galaxyfoods.com;
 www.gqlaxyfoods.com

 In western Canada, the distributor is:
  Sunrise Tofu
  765 Powell St.
  Vancouver, B.C., V6A 1H5.
  604-254-8888.
 In eastern Canada, contact:
  Timbuktu in Markham, Ontario (905-477-7755),
  or Koyo Foods in Montreal, PQ (514-744-1299).

Mail-Order Sources for Marmite and Vegemite, Beans, Grains, Flours, International Condiments and Seasonings, Vinegars, etc.

Cardullo's Gourmet Shop
6 Brattle St.
Cambridge, MA 02138

G.B. Ratto & Co.
821 Washington St.
Oakland, CA. 94607
1-800-325-3483
In California: 1-800-228-3515

In Canada:
Choices Market
2627 W. 16th Ave.,
Vancouver, B.C., Canada V6K 3C2
Phone; (604)736-0009
Fax: (604)736-0011
Natural foods, soyfoods, allergy products, ethnic foods, spices, organic foods, vegan products. No catalog, but will take phone or fax orders and ship COD anywhere in Canada. Prepaid and credit cards accepted. Discounts on volume buying. Friendly service.

Mail-Order Sources for Soyfoods, Vegetarian Foods

ABC Vegetarian Foods
(meat analogs, agar, kosher gelatin, etc.)
Call this toll-free number to order, or to find their nearest location:
1-800-765-6955 (also good for Canada)

The Mail Order Catalog for Healthy Eating
P.O. Box 180
Summertown TN 38483
1-800-695-2241; Fax (931) 964-2291
www.healthy-eating.com
e-mail: catalog@usit.net
Textured soy protein products (including organic), soymilk and soymilk beverage powder, soy protein isolate, silken tofu, Soymage Parmesan, soynut butter, tempeh starter, tofu scrambler mixes, instant gluten powder, nutritional yeast, organic flaxseed, powdered egg replacer, vegetarian Worchestershire sauce, soyfoods cookbooks.

In Canada, see Choices Market, above.

Index

Purchase these cookbooks at your local natural foods
store or book store, or you may order directly from:
Book Publishing Company
P.O. Box 99
Summertown, TN 38483
Please include $3 shipping per book

Also by Bryanna Clark Grogan

Nonna's Italian Kitchen
A tour of regional Italian dishes that
reveals how Italian cooks work their culinary magic. All vegetarian, dairy- and egg-
free. 256 pp $14.95

20 Minutes to Dinner
Get in and out of the kitchen fast
with tempting and nutritious
meat-, egg-, and dairy-free recipes.
192 pp $12.95

The Almost No-Fat Cookbook
Dozens of recipes for winning your family
over to healthful, low-fat eating. 192 pp
$12.95

The Almost No-Fat Holiday Cookbook
Satisfying, festive meals that are
heart-healthy and easy on the
waistline. 192 pp $12.95